TEACH YOURSELF BOOKS

ALTERNATIVE
MEDICINE

ALTERNATIVE
MEDICINE

Loulou Brown

TEACH YOURSELF BOOKS

For UK order queries: please contact Bookpoint Ltd, 39 Milton Park, Abingdon, Oxon OX14 4TD. Telephone: (44) 01235 400414, Fax: (44) 01235 400454. Lines are open from 9.00–6.00, Monday to Saturday, with a 24 hour message answering service. Email address: orders@bookpoint.co.uk

For U.S.A. & Canada order queries: please contact NTC/Contemporary Publishing, 4255 West Touhy Avenue, Lincolnwood, Illinois 60646–1975, U.S.A. Telephone: (847) 679 5500, Fax: (847) 679 2494.

Long renowned as the authoritative source for self-guided learning – with more than 30 million copies sold worldwide – the *Teach Yourself* series includes over 200 titles in the fields of languages, crafts, hobbies, business and education.

A catalogue record for this title is available from The British Library.

Library of Congress Catalog Card Number: On file

First published in UK 1999 by Hodder Headline Plc, 338 Euston Road, London, NW1 3BH.

First published in US 1999 by NTC/Contemporary Publishing, 4255 West Touhy Avenue, Lincolnwood (Chicago), Illinois 60646–1975 U.S.A.

The 'Teach Yourself' name and logo are registered trade marks of Hodder & Stoughton Ltd.

Copyright © 1999 Loulou Brown

In UK: All rights reserved. No part of this publication may be reproduced or transmitted in any form or by any means, electronic or mechanical, including photocopy, recording, or any information storage and retrieval system, without permission in writing from the publisher or under licence from the Copyright Licensing Agency Limited. Further details of such licences (for reprographic reproduction) may be obtained from the Copyright Licensing Agency Limited, of 90 Tottenham Court Road, London W1P 9HE.

In US: All rights reserved. No part of this book may be reproduced, stored in a retrieval system, or transmitted in any form, or by any means, electronic, mechanical, photocopying, or otherwise, without prior permission of NTC/Contemporary Publishing Company.

Cover photo from Barbara Bellingham

Typeset by Transet Limited, Coventry, England.
Printed in Great Britain for Hodder & Stoughton Educational, a division of Hodder Headline Plc, 338 Euston Road, London NW1 3BH by Cox & Wyman Ltd, Reading, Berkshire.

Impression number	10 9 8 7 6 5 4 3 2 1
Year	2004 2003 2002 2001 2000 1999

CONTENTS

Acknowledgements ix
Part I Introduction 1
What is alternative medicine? 3
   Orthodox and holistic approaches to medicine 3
Alternative therapies in the West 5
   Reasons for the growth in alternative medicine 7
Learning about the basics 9
   Helping yourself to health 9
   Buying remedies over the counter 9
   What you can't do for yourself 10
   'Natural' medicines 11
   Importance of a fully qualified reputable therapist 12
Benefits 13
   Positive approach 13
   Respect for the whole individual 13
   Less drastic treatment than orthodox medicine 13
Cautions 14
   Lack of proof of effectiveness of treatment 14
   Problems best treated by orthodox medicine 14
Staying healthy with the right therapy 15
   Consideration of lifestyle 15
When there is a problem 17
   Choosing the appropriate therapy 17
   Finding the right therapist 19
   Considering the cost 20
   Keeping your doctor informed 20
   Possible conflict with orthodox practitioner 20
   Therapies for problems of every age and either sex 21

Part II The Therapies — 25

Part III List of problems and therapies for treatment — 145

Part IV Useful information — 155

National Organizations — 157
General — 157
Acupressure — 161
Acupuncture — 161
Alexander Technique — 163
Anthroposophical medicine — 165
Aromatherapy — 165
Art therapy — 167
Autogenic training — 168
Autosuggestion — 168
Ayurveda — 168
Bates method for better eyesight — 169
Bioenergetics — 170
Biofeedback training — 170
Buteyko method — 171
Chiropractic — 171
Colour therapy — 173
Crystal and gem therapies — 173
Dance therapy — 173
Feldenkrais method — 174
Flotation therapy — 174
Flower remedies — 175
Healing — 175
Hellerwork — 176
Herbal medicine – Chinese — 176
Herbal medicine – Western — 177
Homoeopathy — 178
Hydrotherapy — 179
Hypnotherapy — 180
Iridology — 181
Kinesiology — 182
Light therapy — 183
Massage — 183

Medical astrology _____ 185
Meditation _____ 185
Metamorphic technique _____ 186
Music therapy _____ 186
Naturopathy _____ 187
Osteopathy _____ 188
Pilates _____ 189
Polarity therapy _____ 190
Psychodrama _____ 190
Qigong (Chi kung) _____ 191
Radionics _____ 192
Reflexology _____ 192
Reiki _____ 194
Rolfing _____ 196
Shiatsu _____ 197
Sound therapy _____ 198
T'ai chi _____ 198
Traditional Chinese Medicine _____ 199
Trager bodywork _____ 201
Visualization _____ 201
Yoga _____ 201

Further reading _____ 204
Index _____ 206

For Elisabeth, who has made this a very much better book than it would have been without her help.

CAUTION

In the hands of an experienced practitioner some alternative therapies can be used to treat serious illnesses. They should never be used in this way by anyone else. Self-diagnosis and treatment should only be used for the most minor of ailments and a doctor should be consulted immediately if symptoms persist or become aggravated. Other symptoms such as high or low temperature, delirium or any other indication that the illness is anything more than a minor complaint should be reported to a doctor immediately.

ACKNOWLEDGEMENTS

I would like to acknowledge the following for helping me to produce this book.

First and foremost, I thank my friend Elisabeth Brooke, a member of the National Institute of Medical Herbalists and graduate of Psychosynthesis and Educational Trust, who has accumulated a vast amount of knowledge about many alternative therapies. I don't think I could have managed to write this book without her expert knowledge and advice which she has so generously given me.

I want to thank the following who have provided information and advice, some of whom have checked what I have written: Avigail Ben-Ari, Pilates teacher, Christina Cunliffe, McTimoney Chiropractor, Hermione Gowland and Nigel Gowland for information about alternative medicine in South Africa, Nicola Hall, Chairman of the British Reflexology Association, Annette Middleton, homoeopath, Tracey Khan, aromatherapist, Hilary King, a teacher of the Alexander Technique, Sylvia Leach for information about alternative medicine in Australia, David Repard, Director of the Confederation of Healing Organizations, Linda Seeley, chiropractor, Robin Shepherd, osteopath and the General Osteopathic Council, Mr Gopi Warrier and the Association of Accredited Ayurvedic Practitioners.

Thanks to my friend Alexa Stace for checking and where possible eliminating my deathless prose.

Thanks to Joanne Osborn of Hodder and Stoughton for being so patient about the considerable delay in delivery of the typescript of this book.

Last but not least I want to thank my husband, Bradley Brown, who has diligently searched the internet for information relevant to this book, particularly addresses, phone numbers, faxes and email addresses.

Every effort has been made to contact the holders of copyright material but if any have been inadvertently overlooked, the publisher will be pleased to make the necessary alterations at the first opportunity.

Part I
INTRODUCTION

This book is a practical guide to alternative therapies. There are four parts. The first outlines the basic principles of alternative medicine and describes the present situation regarding alternative therapies in Western countries. Reasons are suggested for the phenomenal growth in alternative medicine as a whole during the last 20 years. The advantages and disadvantages of using alternative therapies are outlined, as are how to prevent ill health and what to do if there is a problem. The second part provides a detailed description of the therapies listed in alphabetical order. The third section consists of a list of conditions and suggested therapies to be used for treatment while the fourth contains a detailed address list of national organizations and a book list for further reading.

What is alternative medicine?

Orthodox and holistic approaches to medicine

Alternative medicine is based on holistic principles. To explain them it may help to compare the orthodox and holistic approaches.

Conventional medicine is based on very detailed and specific scientific knowledge. It adheres to the reductionist principle that for every disease, no matter who has it, there is only one cause and one correct way of dealing with it. Health is seen as simply an absence of symptoms, and ill-health as a malfunction in the body or mind system that has to be corrected and put right by management or manipulation. The emphasis is on fighting, conquering and destroying disease with the use of drugs, surgery or sometimes hard treatment of the mind. In addition, the mind and body are seen as separate entities and are treated by different disciplines, while the spirit is ignored. The focus is on symptoms of disease and it is the symptoms that will be treated while other needs of the person will be largely ignored: needs such as help to cope with fear, depression, anxiety, for example. An imbalance in the relationship between doctor and patient may be created. The doctor is assumed to have knowledge of a patient's disease while the patient may remain ignorant of his or her own problem, with all power and responsibility being handed over to the doctor.

Holistic medicine aims to deal with the patient as a whole, not merely with physical symptoms. Holistic practitioners are concerned to ensure continuing good health and preventing problems that might occur, as well as treating illness. They assume a person exists on many levels and take into account not only the body but also the mind and spirit (the animating or vital principle) of an individual. The mind and spirit are not seen simply as part of the body; each is considered to be a complete system, constantly interacting with one another and of equal importance. The three systems, that is, mind, body and spirit, can be said to be integrated principles of the whole.

Holistic practitioners believe the mind, body and spirit of an individual tend naturally towards a state of balance, known in the West as homeostasis, and that each has a capacity for self-regulation. Equilibrium, however, may be upset by undue emphasis being placed on one part of the whole, and this will affect the other parts. For example, prolonged stress may unbalance the mind and cause the body to react with various symptoms, such as pain or fatigue. The spirit, too, may become unbalanced and depression may occur.

Holistic practitioners tend to focus on the underlying cause rather than on symptoms of an ailment. They want to know why disease – dis-ease as they see it – occurs, with the implication of an underlying lack of balance and disharmony. When there is a problem, the practitioner's function is to work closely with the individual on a long-term basis to help achieve a healthy body, mind and spirit and to promote self-healing. It is the individual, not the practitioner, who is seen as the prime healer, who is actively involved in healing with the help of a remedy or some form of mechanical treatment. The latter are perceived as aids to healing, not cures. Any treatment provided aims to stimulate and support the healing process towards equilibrium rather than heal directly.

Because of the emphasis on the uniqueness of the individual, holistic practitioners do not think diagnosis can be standardized. Often, two people who have previously received orthodox treatment and have been diagnosed with the same disease will receive different treatment from the same alternative practitioner. For instance, a herbalist or homoeopath may give two individuals two completely different remedies for what appears to be the same problem exhibiting similar symptoms.

Holistic practitioners would almost certainly suggest that drugs to control symptoms would not be able to deal with the underlying disturbances that are creating these symptoms. They believe that not only do drugs prevent elimination of impurities but that they might add to the toxins already prevalent. Surgery is thought to destroy homeostasis and is seen as necessary only in the last resort. While it is accepted that a bacterium or virus may trigger an illness, it is thought there is probably a state of susceptibility to disease already prevalent in the individual owing to an imbalance in the mind, which cannot be treated with surgery.

It is important to note that orthodox medicine as practised by many doctors may also be holistic and that there are some (though not many) alternative practitioners who adhere more to the tenets of conventional medicine than to holistic principles. The nature of the therapy does not determine whether or not a practitioner is holistic.

Alternative therapies in the West

Alternative therapies come from all over the world. Some, such as Ayurveda, from India, acupressure, acupuncture and Chinese herbal medicine from China, known collectively as Traditional Chinese Medicine (TCM), and Western herbal medicine (from Europe), are ancient traditional practices that have either re-emerged or have become known and recognized practices in the West. Others, such as homoeopathy from Germany and osteopathy from the USA, originated over a hundred years ago. Many more alternative therapies such as aromatherapy (from France), Bach flower remedies (from England) and biofeedback (from the USA) have been developed over a number of decades during the twentieth century.

Until about the mid-1970s alternative therapies were collectively known as 'fringe' and labelled unconventional or unorthodox practices. Later, the term 'alternative' was applied. In some countries today, such as Australia and the UK, the word 'complementary' is used to describe many therapies that are outside the aegis of orthodox medicine. Alternative, however, embraces all practices that are not orthodox and it is the word used to describe therapies that are not part of conventional medical practice in the USA. It has therefore been decided to use the word alternative rather than complementary throughout this book.

The present position of alternative therapies in some English-speaking countries in the West is described below:

Australia

About half the total population of Australia is reckoned to use at least one non-medically prescribed remedy each year and one-quarter of the total population consult an alternative therapist. Medicare, the medical insurance scheme available throughout Australia, reimburses chiropractic and osteopathic fees as these therapies are state registered in all states and practitioners have to undergo a four-year training at university level. Other therapies are outside the law but tolerated. The Therapeutic Goods Act set up a licensing system for traditional remedies that are allowed to be handled only by certified practitioners. Needles have to be sterilized. It is not permitted to treat certain diseases, such as cancer, by any alternative therapy. The three most popular therapies are probably massage (used a great deal for sports injuries), naturopathy and Chinese and Western herbal medicine.

New Zealand

Like physiotherapists, chiropractors and osteopaths in New Zealand are registered as medical auxiliaries. All other alternative therapies are not registered but operate under common law. Some alternative medicine is taught in medical schools.

South Africa

An Act in 1982 in South Africa incorporated all alternative practitioners into a register supervised by the Associated Health Service Professions Board. It has the same status as the orthodox practitioners' register. There is an obligatory six-year training in alternative medicine, which for the first four years is almost the same as that of medical training. Practitioners specialize in their chosen therapy during the final two years and are not allowed to treat any other therapy than that which they have chosen to practise. Thus, for instance, a homoeopath may provide homoeopathic treatment and prescribe homoeopathic remedies but may not prescribe herbal remedies, while a naturopath may prescribe naturopathic treatment but not homoeopathic remedies. Many practitioners in South Africa consider the system unfortunate as it not only limits the practitioner who is forced to specialize but runs counter to the holistic and inclusive ethos described above.

UK

In the UK chiropractic and osteopathy are registered therapies and only members of the registering boards are allowed to practise. Art and drama therapies are registered as professions supplementary to medicine, which means they receive their patients after diagnosis has been made by a doctor. Otherwise, practitioners of almost any therapy have the right to practise under common law as and when they wish, except they cannot be involved with dentistry, midwifery, veterinary surgery or treat venereal disease. No treatments or remedies for cancer can be advertised but anyone is allowed to treat the disease.

Roughly one-third of the total adult population use an alternative therapy at least once a year and currently (1999) there are over four million visits a year to alternative practitioners. Usage of alternative therapies doubled between the years 1986 and 1991 and the number of practitioners is currently increasing at the rate of 11 per cent per annum. It is estimated that three-quarters of the GP fundholding practices would like to see alternative therapies available on the NHS. In 1995 a Consumers' Association survey showed healing, osteopathy, chiropractic, homoeopathy, aromatherapy and acupuncture to be the most popular alternative therapies, while aromatherapy is the fastest growing therapy.

USA

In the USA each of the 50 states decides its own policy regarding alternative medicine. In most states alternative techniques are described as medical practices. Some states have introduced regulatory laws. Chiropractic, the most popular alternative therapy, is registered by all states and doctors refer to and receive referrals from chiropractors. (Osteopathy has for some time been considered part of orthodox medical practice.) In some states, acupuncture can be practised only by physicians, while other states allow the therapy to be practised by non-medical practitioners. Naturopathic medicine is recognized and licensed in ten states, while herbal medicine is banned in many states. New York State, however, recognizes all therapies and supports freedom of choice in health care. Ayurveda, chiropractic and TCM are very popular therapies, aromatherapy and homoeopathy less so. Medical students take courses in alternative medicine at over 30 medical schools.

Very nearly half the total population of the USA use at least one form of alternative medicine every year and more visits are made to alternative practitioners than to conventional doctors. Several health insurers now cover some alternative therapies if they are recommended to do so by the patient's doctor.

Reasons for the growth in alternative medicine

During the last 20 years, and particularly during the 1990s, the growth of alternative therapies in the West has been remarkable. This has been due to a number of factors.

- The very great advances in medicine and general public health throughout the twentieth century have meant that people in Western countries no longer have to be solely preoccupied with survival. Health is perceived to be not merely the absence of disease but a positive quality of living.
- Patients demand to be more actively involved in, and knowledgeable about, their own health care rather than dependent on their doctors and ignorant about their own bodies, minds and symptoms of disease.
- There is a fear of conventional drug treatment and surgery. This fear is not perceived by doctors to be a problem that requires alleviating.
- Patients are becoming aware of the limitations of orthodox medicine. The following two examples may illustrate the extent of these limitations. In the UK in 1994, a report by Dr Chris Worth, Director of Public Health, Western Yorkshire Health Authority, stated that one in four patients suffered a deleterious condition as a direct or indirect result of medical treatment, and that one in ten hospital outpatient admissions represented conditions arising as a result of treatment. In late 1998, a UK report by the British National Formulary suggested that doctors are writing about 30 million prescriptions per year for drugs that may not be suitable for their patients, either because they do not work, have dangerous side-effects or because there may be no better medicine on the market.
- Patients want more communication with, and more information from, their doctors than they receive. They also want relief from stress, anxiety and worries that may appear to be unrelated to the problems they have come to their doctors about. They find they can communicate with, and receive more information from, holistic alternative practitioners who are prepared to spend much more time talking to patients about their perceived needs. It is estimated that on average alternative therapists spend eight times as long on each consultation than doctors do.

Learning about the basics

Helping yourself to health

If you are treated by an orthodox practitioner you may be expected to remain a passive recipient of treatment; the word 'patient' implies passivity. You may be given treatment to eliminate symptoms but may not be expected to do much about your illness or to question why you are ill. You only go to a doctor if you are ill. The notion of going to a doctor if you are in good health is absurd.

An alternative therapist, however, will almost certainly expect you (who might be called a client, pupil or student rather than patient) to take an active part in your treatment by, for instance, thinking carefully about why you are ill, and whether your lifestyle might have created a problem. You may even be asked to help decide what sort of treatment you require. A reputable practitioner will regard you as an equal, not a subordinate, and you will be expected to share in the decision-making process.

You will be expected to help yourself. This means you will be expected to take charge of your health, which may mean a great deal of change. A responsible therapist will help you to recognize many problems that are caused by poor living habits and self abuse. If you smoke you will almost certainly have been told by your orthodox practitioner that it makes sense to give up and all reputable alternative therapists will also encourage you to stop. It also helps to cut down on alcohol. Stimulants and tranquillizers may help you through the days and nights but they will harm your health in the long term. In almost all cases your weight can be controlled by eating moderately and keeping to a sensible diet. Try to see such suggestions as a positive challenge. You will probably be encouraged to see your therapist at regular intervals, say, once every six months, for a check-up to prevent sickness and ensure your continued good health.

Buying remedies over the counter

During the last ten years there has been a massive increase in alternative remedies that can be bought over the counter in both reputable and more dubious stores. These are usually in the form of tinctures, tablets or creams and may be, for example, Ayurvedic, flower, herbal, homoeopathic or nutritional remedies or supplements. Here it is important to reiterate that alternative therapies treat the whole person, not simply symptoms of disease. Each person is treated as someone unique with a unique problem. Taking remedies to treat symptoms common to everyone is adopting the ethos of orthodox medicine and runs contrary to that of alternative medicine.

Nevertheless, it is unreasonable to expect anyone to go to either a doctor or alternative therapist for a minor complaint. In any event it is reckoned that just over 75 per cent of health problems are dealt with by either self care or by doing nothing at all. Also, it does seem that some remedies bought over the counter are very effective in alleviating particular problems, at least short term. The Bach rescue remedy, for example, has proved extremely beneficial. Don't, however, expect miracles or immediate results and do think about what you are buying, why you are buying it and the recommended dosage to take. The following points may be useful to note:

- Always check that a remedy is suitable before you buy it. Read the label or ask the pharmacist.
- If you are taking other medicines do *not* buy over-the-counter remedies.
- Make sure you store your remedies properly. Always store them in the container you purchase them in. Make sure the lids are closed securely.
- Always store remedies out of the reach of children.
- See your doctor or alternative therapist if your symptoms do not clear or become more severe.

What you can't do for yourself

You cannot ensure that your problem will be eliminated; that is not the way alternative therapies work. An alternative therapy may be able to alleviate and even clear a problem but it will not be able to effect a cure. If you go to an alternative practitioner, he or she will want to find out the root cause of the symptom or symptoms you are experiencing. This may not be easy because the symptoms may not be displaying an obvious problem. To take an extreme example, if you go to an Alexander teacher or chiropractor with a bad back and stooped shoulders, you will probably be judged to have poor posture. You will certainly be helped to alleviate the pain in the back and to correct your poor posture but the underlying problem may take some time to unearth. It may be, for example, that you are unconsciously defending yourself against a fearful attack upon your person because as a child you were physically abused by one of your parents. You may have put this horror out of your mind and now firmly refuse to accept that anything untoward happened in your childhood. It may take a long time with a lot of therapy – perhaps several alternative therapies may be required – for you to accept what happened long ago. Once you acknowledge what has happened, however, you can really begin to change. You can not only change your posture so your back doesn't hurt any more, but you can enhance your self-esteem and change what are probably negative thoughts about yourself and your life into positive ones. This is an extreme instance of repression; most problems do not have such a very serious underlying cause. It is, however, meant to illustrate that you have to learn to accept that time is needed for both diagnosis and treatment.

'Natural' medicines

There is a belief that alternative therapies are natural, in tune with nature, and that because they are less mechanistic than orthodox medicine they are automatically safe and do not interfere either with our minds or bodies. This, however, is a false assumption. Therapies such as homoeopathy and Chinese and Western herbalism use oral medicinal remedies; others such as massage are physically manipulative; yet others such as hypnotherapy, visualization and biofeedback manipulate the mind. All such therapies interfere with the existing balance in the mind, body and spirit. It may be the aim is to enable the homeostatic processes of the body to function properly again to create harmony and balance, nevertheless there is interference. In the wrong hands, such interference may prove to be of no benefit and may cause harm.

If you are treated properly by a fully qualified and competent practitioner there is almost no possibility of you coming to any harm. The problem is that almost all alternative therapies, apart from osteopathy and chiropractic, are unregulated in most English-speaking countries. This means that anyone can set up as, say, an Ayurvedic practitioner, an aromatherapist, a homoeopath, a herbalist or a masseur without adequate training and without being registered by a governing body. It is essential you find qualified practitioners through reputable national organizations.

Importance of a fully qualified reputable therapist

For any therapy, it is essential to find a reputable, fully qualified therapist, otherwise you will not benefit from the treatment provided and you may come to harm. It is best to contact a national organization rather than rely on friends or advertisements. Before making an appointment with a therapist, check the following details:

- The therapist's qualifications.
- How long has the therapist been in practice?
- What sort of training has the therapist had, and for how long did the training last?
- Is the therapist registered with a recognized professional organization?
- Does the organization have a code of practice?
- Ask about the possible length of a course of treatment (though to be fair this may be impossible to estimate).
- Ask about any side-effects of the treatment.
- Ask about the cost.

After your first visit to a therapist, ask yourself the following questions:

- Did you find the therapist easy to talk to?
- Did you find the therapist's conduct entirely professional?
- Did you find you were listened to?
- Did the therapist ask about your lifestyle, work, moods, etc?
- Did you think you received a clear, comprehensible diagnosis?
- Did you feel safe with the treatment given or prescribed?
- Did you have everything clearly and properly explained?
- Did you feel you had an empathy with and trusted the therapist?
- Did you feel you were given enough time to explain your problem and absorb the information given to you?
- Did you consider the cost of the treatment reasonable?

If you answer 'yes' to at least eight of these questions you have probably found a therapist who will treat you well. If not, find another therapist.

Benefits

Positive approach

Alternative practitioners focus on good health and prevention of disease. They operate a health-orientated care system rather than a disease-orientated cure system like orthodox practitioners. They see their role as helping their patients to develop their well-being and enjoy their lives.

You will be encouraged to become responsible for your health to enable you to discipline your life against self abuse in the form of poor diet, stress, anxiety, etc, and to evaluate your moral and ethical standards of living in order to aim for happiness, contentment, hope, love and joy. Your practitioner will help you to decide how you intend to do this. He or she will act as a guide, facilitator or teacher who is concerned with your long-term development.

Respect for the whole individual

Alternative therapists regard each individual as unique. They see problems that are the result of unique external circumstances and constitutional differences, in addition to the presenting symptoms. When you visit an alternative practitioner all aspects of yourself will be taken into account, as well as the symptoms of your problem. You will be seen as a human being with a unique lifestyle, attitudes, tastes, stresses and relationships. You will be encouraged to discuss matters you may normally not talk about with your doctor, such as emotional stresses and strains, your work, sexual relationships, relationships with your parents and your medical history. You will be encouraged to talk about your aims in life, what really matters to you, your interests, particularly issues you are involved in creatively. You will be given time to talk so that your therapist can assess your needs and any underlying problems. In short, you will be treated with respect and not simply as a body with a symptom.

Less drastic treatment than orthodox medicine

An alternative therapist recognizes that your feelings, anxieties and fears as a patient, as well as his or her own, are significant for your joint relationship. Emphasis is placed on a healthy lifestyle, positive attitudes, happy disposition and prevention of disease. Treatment, in the form of, for example, exercise, massage, manipulation and remedies, focuses on health rather than disease. It is far less drastic than orthodox medicine.

Cautions

Lack of proof of effectiveness of treatment

There has been very little scientific research conducted on alternative therapies to prove their effectiveness. This is partly because of the understandable antipathy of some orthodox practitioners who are not prepared to fund investigations of therapies that are a potential threat to their profession. It is also partly because alternative practitioners are reluctant to use scientific methods that are for the most part alien to the basic principles of holistic medicine. Also, there are many therapies such as healing, radionics and homoeopathy that are impossible to quantify using scientific methods. Even so, the small body of research that has been undertaken has come up with some very positive results. For instance, during the last 30 years, scientific research, particularly with regard to biofeedback (see p. 50) has shown that to a significant extent the mind can control physiological processes that previously were regarded by orthodox practitioners to be wholly automatic, that is, responses of the autonomic nervous system. Today, far more respect is accorded by orthodox practitioners to mind–body therapies such as meditation and yoga. It has been found that certain emotional attitudes result in specific physical postures, gestures or facial expressions, and it is beginning to be accepted that exercise and manipulative therapies such as the Alexander Technique, chiropractic, osteopathy, Pilates and Rolfing can induce psychological well-being by bringing the musculoskeletal structure of the physical body back into balance, thus reversing processes that have given rise to what bioenergetic practitioners term 'body armouring'.

Problems best treated by orthodox medicine

There are many problems, particularly accidents in the form of structural damage, burns and infectious diseases, that orthodox medicine can both diagnose and treat far more efficiently and effectively than any alternative therapy. There are some people who say they would rather die than be treated by an orthodox practitioner, but if they suffered a life-threatening illness, would they not rather visit a doctor, be diagnosed, treated with drugs or operated on in hospital with a view to being cured, rather than continue without any treatment, possibly in great pain, with a short expectation of life? Invasive diseases such as cancer are perhaps symptomatic of some other underlying problem that requires attending to with less invasive means. If left untreated, however, the severe symptoms could and probably would prove fatal. They have to be eliminated as soon as possible. There are also accidents that involve broken bones or third-degree burns, or high fevers caused by viruses, all of which require immediate treatment by a doctor.

There are some alternative therapies, for example, acupressure, aromatherapy and reflexology, that have proved to be extremely beneficial in alleviating the stress and anxiety associated with surgery, or the severe side-effects caused by some drugs. Healing can take place much faster than would have been the case without such alternative treatments, which do not affect or counteract the oral medication.

Staying healthy with the right therapy

Consideration of lifestyle

Most alternative therapists will ask you about your lifestyle. This is an umbrella term that includes, for example, whether you are male or female, how old you are, where you live, whom you live with, what people are important to you, whether or not you have children, what your work is, what your interests are, what your aims are in life, what sort of food you eat, whether you drink alcohol, smoke, or take drugs socially. The questions asked may well seem intrusive, but bear in mind that the therapist is looking to treat the whole of you, your mind, body and spirit, not simply your symptoms. It is very important you feel empathy for and trust your therapist well enough to be able to answer the questions asked as thoroughly and as honestly as you can.

It is important to realize that you have to learn to work actively to achieve a lifestyle that will maintain health and prevent illness. There are a number of ways in which you can help yourself without seeing a therapist.

- *Healthy eating.* Few people in English-speaking Western countries enjoy food; most gulp down fast food for fodder. But taking time to prepare and eat good food can be a pleasurable and enjoyable activity, and this is essential for good health. Think about what food you eat, and eat well. You need to consume lots of fruit and vegetables, preferably organic, wholegrains, nuts, oily fish and white meat. At the same time you might consider cutting down your consumption of red meat and dairy products such as milk, butter and cheese. Cut back on your consumption of alcohol and stop smoking. You know it makes sense. For further advice about diet and healthy eating, seek the advice of a naturopath (see Part II).

- *Exercise.* Most of us, including children, are not getting enough exercise. We need to get out of our houses, work places and cars and walk more. A brisk walk for 20 minutes three times a week that makes you sweat a bit will keep you in trim. If you live in an area that is unsuitable to walk in or you dislike the activity, take up a sport. Or you might want to consider an exercise such as qigong or t'ai chi (see Part II for a description of the therapies). These activities are suitable for everyone from early childhood to old age. Exercise improves mood, helps to lift depression and may even boost self-esteem.

- *Sleep.* We need plenty of sleep. Very probably you are not getting enough of it. One hundred years ago when the pace of life was much slower, people slept an average of nine hours each night. Today the average is somewhat less than eight. Many of us only manage to sleep six hours or less. Quite apart from tiredness, lack of sleep causes depression, tenseness, anxiety, headaches, lack of self-esteem and a host of other physical and mental symptoms. Aim for eight hours. If you suffer from insomnia do some breathing and relaxation exercises (see Part II).

- *Controlling emotions.* We have to learn to cope with negative emotions such as anxiety, depression and loneliness, grief, anger, sadness, jealousy, disappointment and fears that affect the immune system, reducing antibody production. Depression, for example, is associated with suppressed immune responses. Unconscious attitudes, too, may have a great deal to do with the conditions that give rise to disease; changing them can only be achieved if they become conscious. Not surprisingly, research has shown that people who are happy and optimistic about their lives tend to be healthier than those who are depressed and miserable. To help cope with negative emotions, try some art therapy, music therapy, visualization, meditation or yoga (see Part II for a description of the therapies).

■ *Managing stress*. The way we live in 'developed' societies is stressful: living in overcrowded towns and cities fearful of violence, with traffic jams and long hours of repetitive work, living with too many people or living alone ... the list is endless. It is true that a little short-term stress may be beneficial. Stress stimulates, creates a buzz and concentrates the mind. With long-term stress, however, problems start to occur. Concentration may start to lapse, and we may become aggressive and irritable and suffer an inability to sleep for long periods. Physical symptoms may start to appear, such as back and neck aches, diarrhoea, dry mouth, fatigue, headaches, heartburn, indigestion, migraines, palpitations, skin problems and sweating. Studies have linked stress to colds and cold sores.

We need to be able to manage stress and there are many therapies that can help. Even babies can get stressed. If this is the case, give your baby a gentle massage all over the body. Babies love being touched by their mothers, and their fathers too, if they know them well. If your baby's stress is severe, go to an osteopath who is an expert in cranial osteopathy. Techniques used in this therapy are so gentle they will not harm your baby and may be very beneficial. You might think about giving yourself a treat and having an aromatherapy or Swedish massage, some lessons in the Alexander Technique or float in a flotation tank. Or, to save spending money, try some relaxation and breathing (see Part II for a description of the therapies).

When there is a problem

Choosing the appropriate therapy

If you have decided to try an alternative therapy it is important you find the right therapy for your problem. This book aims to help you find it. More often than not, you will find you have a choice. Quite apart from choosing a therapy suitable for treating your problem, you will want to choose a therapy you think you might like. In Part II 53 therapies are listed in alphabetical order for easy access. To help you to choose a therapy with which you may feel comfortable, the therapies are listed below in categories:

Creative therapies

Art therapy
Colour therapy
Dance therapy
Music therapy
Psychodrama
Sound therapy

Exercise therapies

Alexander Technique
Bates method
Bioenergetics
Breathing and relaxation
Buteyko method
Feldenkrais method
Pilates
Qigong
T'ai chi
Yoga

Manipulative and touch therapies

Acupressure
Aromatherapy
Chiropractic
Hellerwork
Kinesiology
Massage
Metamorphic technique
Osteopathy
Polarity therapy
Reflexology
Reiki
Rolfing
Shiatsu
Trager bodywork

Mind and spirit therapies

Autogenic training
Autosuggestion
Biofeedback training
Biorhythms
Healing
Hypnotherapy
Medical astrology
Meditation
Radionics
Visualization

Oral therapies

Chinese herbal medicine
Flower remedies
Homoeopathy
Naturopathy
Western herbal medicine

Water therapies

Flotation therapy
Hydrotherapy

There are others that do not fit into any of the above categories. They are:

Acupuncture
Anthroposophical medicine
Ayurveda
Crystal and gem therapies
Iridology
Light therapy

INTRODUCTION 19

It may help to note that, very broadly speaking, there are some therapies that have been taken up more by men than women. These tend to be manipulative practices such as chiropractic, Hellerwork, osteopathy and Trager bodywork. In the main such therapies are more respected by orthodox practitioners and are closer in outlook to orthodox medicine, perhaps because they appear to be more scientific. There are others that are much more gentle, sensuous, touching and feeling in their approach, such as aromatherapy, colour therapy, flower remedies, healing, massage, music therapy and reflexology. These have been taken up more by women. (It is interesting to note that in the UK aromatherapy, massage and reflexology are available in 90 per cent of palliative care settings, that is, AIDS and cancer. Nurses are particularly keen on aromatherapy and reflexology.)

If you find you cannot make up your mind by reading about what is available in books or by talking to other people, the best way to choose a therapy is to try out several therapies and make your choice, that is, if you can afford to do so. Quite a few therapies are available in short introductory group sessions at, for example, health centres, and run for a day or for several hours each week for a month or so. These are usually reasonably priced and will give you a good idea of what you might expect.

It is important you choose the therapy you want. Do not rely on friends, relatives or even the person closest to you to make this choice for you. No one should tell you what therapy to use. It is for you to make the choice.

Finding the right therapist

You have to make sure you find the right therapist. Even though you may have found the therapy appropriate to your problem and one you feel happy with, and have also found a reputable, fully qualified and experienced practitioner who treats your problems well, you still may feel he or she is not right for you. Perhaps there is a lack of empathy or trust or perhaps the treatment is too expensive. Whatever the reason, if you don't feel happy, find another therapist. Sometimes it takes some time to find the right person. Once you do find the right one, you will probably find he or she is qualified in a number of therapies and can treat a number of problems. (Note this is not the case in South Africa – see above.)

Considering the cost

A crucial consideration in deciding whether or not to go to an alternative therapist is the cost. Users of alternative therapies in the West tend to be young, or middle-aged professional people, that is, those who can afford the very considerable cost involved. It is difficult, and in many countries impossible, to get alternative health care free of charge, though the situation is slowly changing for the better in this respect. In the UK, for instance, it is quite possible you may be referred to an alternative practitioner through the National Health Service (NHS), provided you have a GP who is sympathetic to alternative medicine. It is hoped that in the future alternative medicine will be perceived as part of a wide range of health care and that patients will be able to pick and choose the type of health care they prefer, whether allopathic or alternative, and that all types of medicine will be made available at little or no cost. At the moment, however, this is not the case. There are a great many people who might well benefit from alternative medicine but who cannot afford it.

Keeping your doctor informed

It is best to let your doctor know if you are seeing an alternative therapist for treatment of a problem. This is particularly important if you are being treated by your doctor for the same problem and are taking prescribed medication. It is possible your doctor may recommend, or refer you to, an alternative practitioner.

Possible conflict with orthodox practitioner

You have to consider your doctor's reaction to being told you are seeing an alternative practitioner. If you are on good terms you should have no problems. If, on the other hand, you don't know your doctor, or know that he or she may be hostile to alternative medicine, you have an additional problem to deal with. It is always best to keep your doctor informed (see above), but there are circumstances where it might be best not to do this. If you are really worried about your doctor's reaction, maybe you should consider finding another doctor, difficult though this might be, or drop the idea of an alternative therapy.

It is a sad fact that some orthodox practitioners still consider most if not all alternative therapies to be alien and foolish practices. They feel their own profession is under threat from a new, untested and unscientific medicine and most are so hard pressed that they have little time to learn about something different.

You may be told by your doctor that seeing an alternative practitioner would not be beneficial. Don't, however, be led by this negative and authoritative suggestion. It is a matter for you to decide. Make up your own mind. Don't let your doctor make it up for you.

Therapies for problems of every age and either sex

Listed below is a selection of specific problems relating to either men or women or people of either sex at different age groups. For each problem two therapies are suggested that might alleviate and possibly clear it. There may be many more that are suitable. To find out about the therapies, look in the A–Z list in Part II. For a more detailed list of symptoms and remedies see pp. 147–54.

For babies

babies' colic   acupressure, cranial osteopathy
nappy rash   aromatherapy, Western herbal medicine
sleep problems   Bach flower remedies, cranial osteopathy
teething   homoeopathy, Western herbal medicine

For children

bedwetting (enuresis)   chiropractic, cranial osteopathy
chilblains   massage, naturopathy
croup   aromatherapy, homoeopathy
eczema   Chinese herbal medicine, reflexology
glue ear   cranial osteopathy, naturopathy
hyperactivity   breathing and relaxation, naturopathy
impetigo   aromatherapy, naturopathy
stammering   breathing and relaxation, visualization
stye   homoeopathy, naturopathy
temper tantrums   Bach flower remedies, naturopathy
warts   aromatherapy, homoeopathy

For teenagers

acne   aromatherapy, naturopathy
anaemia   aromatherapy, homoeopathy
anorexia nervosa   art therapy, dance therapy

anxiety   aromatherapy, biofeedback
athlete's foot   aromatherapy, Western herbal medicine
bulimia nervosa   aromatherapy, massage
dandruff   massage, naturopathy
hysteria   breathing and relaxation, music therapy
impetigo   aromatherapy, naturopathy
spots and pimples   aromatherapy, naturopathy

For sports people

back problems   Alexander Technique, chiropractic
blisters   aromatherapy, Western herbal medicine
bruises   aromatherapy, homoeopathy
bursitis   hydrotherapy, massage
cramp   massage, yoga
dislocations   chiropractic, osteopathy
muscle pain   hydrotherapy, Rolfing
repetitive strain injury (RSI)   acupressure, massage
sprains   massage, osteopathy
whiplash   chiropractic, osteopathy

For older people

arthritis   acupuncture, naturopathy
constipation   massage, naturopathy
frozen shoulder   chiropractic, massage
fluid retention (oedema)   naturopathy, Western herbal medicine
hardening of the arteries   breathing and relaxation, naturopathy
obesity   hypnotherapy, naturopathy
varicose veins   naturopathy, yoga

For men

baldness (alopecia)   aromatherapy, Western herbal medicine
back pain   acupuncture, chiropractic
impotence   autogenic training, meditation
infertility (male)   autogenic training, naturopathy
neck pain   chiropractic, reflexology
premature ejaculation   Chinese herbal medicine, hypnotherapy
prostate enlargement   naturopathy, yoga
snoring   hypnotherapy, osteopathy

For women

back pain in pregnancy   flotation, osteopathy
breastfeeding – lack of milk   acupressure, Western herbal medicine
cystitis   homoeopathy, naturopathy
endometriosis   Chinese herbal medicine, naturopathy
frigidity   dance therapy, meditation
heavy periods (menorrhagia)   acupuncture, naturopathy
hot flushes   meditation, naturopathy
infertility (female)   hydrotherapy, naturopathy
labour (when in)   acupressure, breathing and relaxation
menstrual pain (dysmenorrhoea)   naturopathy, yoga
morning sickness   acupressure, homoeopathy
post-natal depression   cranial osteopathy, naturopathy
stress incontinence (urine)   hydrotherapy, Pilates
pre-menstrual syndrome (PMS)   Chinese herbal medicine, reflexology
vaginal thrush   hydrotherapy, Western herbal medicine
vaginitis (inflammation of vagina)   aromatherapy, naturopathy

Part II
THE THERAPIES

The therapies are listed in alphabetical order under the following headings:

Definition and principles
Brief outline
Conditions helped
How to find a therapist or teacher
What to expect
Self treatment (only listed if applicable)
Limitations and dangers

Acupressure

Definition and principles

The aim of acupressure, part of Traditional Chinese Medicine (see p. 134), is to balance *Qi* (life energy) through acupuncture points (acupoints) using finger, thumb, feet and knee pressure, and massage. No needles are used; all treatment acts only on the skin.

Brief outline

Acupressure has been practised for at least 3,000 years and is believed to predate acupuncture. It is used in China for treating common ailments and for boosting the body's immune system. Many acupuncturists in the West are now using acupressure as part of their treatment. Studies have shown it relieves nausea caused by anaesthesia, travel sickness and pregnancy.

Conditions helped

There are very many ailments acupressure claims to alleviate and help to clear, particularly the following: addictions, anxiety, arthritis, back pain, catarrh, chilblains, cystitis, depression, diarrhoea, digestive disorders, dizziness, eyestrain, fainting, fatigue, frozen shoulder, headaches, heavy periods, high blood pressure, indigestion, insomnia, joint pains, laryngitis, lumbago, menopausal problems, migraine, morning sickness, nausea, neuralgia, sciatica, sinusitis, stress, sweating, tinnitus, tiredness, toothache, travel sickness, vertigo and vomiting. Acupressure is also used to promote health and general well-being.

How to find a therapist

If you cannot find an acupressure organization, contact one of the national acupuncture organizations listed in Part IV for further information.

What to expect

You will be asked about your medical history and lifestyle and will be diagnosed according to Traditional Chinese Medicine (TCM) methods of diagnosis (see p. 134). You should wear loose-fitting clothes and sit or lie on a raised surface or mat for treatment. You may experience some discomfort when acupoints are pressed.

Self treatment

If you want to use acupressure to treat yourself, the best way is to learn from an experienced practitioner.

Two self-help techniques are outlined below.

- *For sinusitis*: press with the thumb between the eyebrows for one to two minutes.
- *For nausea*: press with the thumb about 50 mm (2 in) from wrist on the underside of the arm for one to two minutes.

Limitations and dangers

Do not use acupressure if you have a serious illness, infection or fever.

Acupuncture

Definition and principles

The word 'acupuncture' means 'pricking with a needle'. Acupuncture treatment aims to restore the balance of the bodily energy or life force, *Qi*, that has been disrupted, to relieve pain and restore health. It is part of TCM (see p. 134).

Brief outline

Acupuncture is an ancient therapy and is known to have been practised in China about 3,500 years ago. The therapy was used extensively in England in the nineteenth century for the relief of pain and fever. Today the treatment is becoming increasingly popular in all English-speaking Western countries.

Conditions helped

There is a very wide range of problems that can be treated by acupuncture. The following conditions have benefited from treatment and are among those most commonly treated by Western acupuncturists: acne, addictions, anorexia nervosa, anxiety, arthritis, asthma, back pain, Bell's palsy, breathlessness, bronchitis, bulimia nervosa, cold sores, common cold, constipation, cystitis, depression, diarrhoea, ear infections, eczema, faecal incontinence, frozen shoulder, hay fever, headaches, heavy periods, high blood pressure, impotence, indigestion, infertility, influenza, insomnia, irregular periods, irritable bowel syndrome (IBS), laryngitis, migraines, neck pain, neuralgia, painful periods, palpitations, peptic ulcers, piles, poor circulation, pre-menstrual syndrome (PMS), psoriasis, rheumatism, sciatica, shock, sinusitis, sports injuries, tinnitus and urinary incontinence. Acupuncture has also been used to alleviate fear and pain in dentistry and childbirth.

How to find a therapist

It is essential you find a reputable and fully qualified acupuncturist. Do not rely on friends or advertisements for a practitioner, rather contact a national organization (see Part IV). Acupuncturists are not necessarily members of professional organizations. If you are treated by an unqualified acupuncturist you will almost certainly gain no benefit from the treatment and may be harmed. It is advisable to ask a practitioner about the length of his or her training. All reputable acupuncturists should have studied for at least four years part-time.

What to expect

At the initial session there will be detailed checks and tests, based on TCM principles (see p. 134), and this may last for up to 90 minutes. Questions will be asked about your medical history, present symptoms, length of illness, whether or not you sleep well, your age and lifestyle, phobias and reactions to stress. The colour, shape and movement of your tongue will be checked as well as your skin texture and colouring, hair texture, posture and movement, breathing, voice and pulse. In order to diagnose any disturbance in the flow of *Qi* and possible disease of internal organs, the acupuncturist will feel your pulse very carefully, using a special method called palpating. (In traditional acupuncture, there are deemed to be 12 pulses, six in each wrist, with each pulse representing one of the 12 main organs.) In addition, the practitioner will assess your spirit or 'vital force' to find out whether or not it is thriving. This requires a close rapport between practitioner and patient for the practitioner to 'see' the spirit and assess its vitality. Emotions are considered to emanate from a person's spirit and acupuncture tries to balance the emotions by making sure there is no extreme emotion and no lack. Following the diagnosis a course of treatment will be proposed. Very roughly, a short course to alleviate and clear a relatively minor problem averages around ten sessions but a severe condition may require up to 100 treatments.

Very fine needles, previously unused or thoroughly sterilized, are inserted into the skin in various parts of the body known as acupoints for up to 30 minutes at a time. If performed correctly this is a very quick, painless and bloodless procedure. You may feel a slight numbness or tingling sensation. This means that the needle has reached the required depth and has touched the flow of *Qi* in the meridian. The sensation indicates that the point has been accurately located. The needles, made from silver or stainless steel, are hardly thicker than head hair, and the number of needles used varies from one to as many as fifteen. They may be left alone or may be stimulated either manually, that is, rotated between the acupuncturist's finger and thumb to call up or disperse the *Qi*, or electronically, by the acupuncturist.

Sometimes a process known as moxibustion may be practised together with acupuncture. The word is derived from the Japanese 'moe gusa' which means 'burning herb'. A 'ma', consisting of dried common mugwort (*Artemisia vulgaris*), may be placed on an acupoint. It is lit and allowed to smoulder slowly until you feel your skin becoming warm. It is then removed. You will probably find this gives you a pleasant, warm sensation. This is used to warm your *Qi*, the energy flow. It is not only beneficial in alleviating symptoms but is likely to help you feel the cold less acutely. Moxibustion is used more in countries that have a cold winter season, such as the UK, Canada, the north of north America, northern China, Korea and Japan. It is particularly indicated if you are deficient in yang, the aspect of yin-yang that is responsible for warmth. Moxibustion can be applied over an area of the body that has become cold, such as a 'frozen' shoulder or painful menstruation. The technique is claimed to be very effective in the treatment of earache and the early stages of ear infections.

After treatment you may feel a certain heaviness of the limbs and pleasantly relaxed. Acute conditions may be treated on a daily basis while chronic problems are usually treated weekly. You are likely to start feeling much better after about five or six treatments. Initially it is possible you may feel a little worse immediately after treatment than you did before it began. This may be a good sign as it shows you are reacting to the treatment. The acupuncturist will probably use fewer needles and for a shorter time at the following session. If there is no improvement after eight sessions it is probable that the cause of the problem has not been diagnosed correctly or that there is a certain factor or factors in the diagnosis which are important but have been ignored. You are advised to stop the treatment and find someone else to treat you, or go to your doctor.

Even though you may be well you will probably be advised to have at least four acupuncture sessions per year to tune the body and maintain good health.

Limitations and dangers

If used correctly acupuncture is not harmful. Note, however, that if needles remain inserted for longer than the body can handle them, granulation tissue may be produced. Also, if needles are reused and have not been sterilized in an autoclave there is a danger of transmission of the HIV virus, Hepatitis C and other life-threatening conditions.

If you are taking prescribed medication it is essential you inform your doctor that you are having acupuncture. It is possible, though unlikely, that acupuncture treatment may interfere with the medication. It is, however, far more likely that any medication will interfere with the very complex and delicate treatment to ensure *Qi* balance within the meridians.

Acupuncture cannot help with conditions where there is a genetic defect (such as muscular dystrophy) or advanced pathological conditions.

Alexander Technique

Definition and principles

The Alexander Technique teaches new ways of thinking about and using our bodies so we can eliminate unconscious habits of tension, particularly those that constrict the spine, thereby improving physical and psychological well-being. A fundamental principle is that the mind and body are interconnected and interact with each other. Practitioners see the technique as a way of living rather than as a therapy, and as a method of promoting well-being through psychophysical re-education rather than as treating dysfunction. They do not profess to treat or claim to cure anything. They refer to themselves as teachers and to those who come to them as pupils, rather than as clients or patients, and do not claim to teach a form of alternative medicine. Pupils are taught to become aware of balance, posture and movement applied to all actions in everyday life, such as thinking, breathing, eating, speaking, walking, reading and lying down.

Brief outline

The Alexander Technique is named after its creator, an Australian born in Tasmania. Frederick Matthias Alexander (1869–1955) trained as an actor. He began to lose his voice on stage. As medical treatment did not help his problem, he decided to help himself. He researched the problem by observing himself many times in front of three-way mirrors and began to realize that his postural habits and bodily movements affected his voice. This was because he was squeezing his vocal cords by pulling his head back and down and shortening his spine. He decided he could cure the problem with his voice by stopping or 'inhibiting' these habits of contraction and noted that the relationship between the head, neck and back was extremely important to the functioning of the whole organism. Once he changed his postural habits and movements his voice improved as well as his breathing and general well-being.

Alexander came to London in 1904 where he was known as the 'breathing man'. Actors and others with respiratory problems came to him for help, and his discoveries became the basis of a technique for retraining the body's movements and positions.

Today the Alexander Technique is taught worldwide, predominantly in Australia, Israel, the UK and USA, as well as in many countries in Europe. Many professional organizations, such as acting or music establishments, encourage their members to have lessons in the technique. Recently there has been growing interest shown by business employers, who are becoming increasingly aware of the need to promote the well-being of their employees to ensure greater productivity. Many recognize that the Alexander Technique can combat the myriad new problems suffered in the workplace as a result of new technology, such as repetitive strain injury (RSI) or new types of back problems.

Conditions helped

The Alexander Technique aims to remove the cause, not the symptoms, of disorders. Nevertheless, pupils very often find there is a reduction, and sometimes disappearance, of disorders after learning the technique. Breathing, circulation, digestion and elimination processes become easier for the body as a result of unrestricted movement and improved tone of muscles. There is thus greater scope for an individual's own curative powers to take effect. There are also many claims that the technique has not only brought about an improvement in people's health but has also contributed towards emotional well-being, mental alertness and resistance to stress.

Teachers and pupils claim the Alexander Technique alleviates the following: anxiety, asthma, back pain, breathing problems, bursitis, depression, exhaustion, gout, gynaecological disorders, headaches, high blood pressure, hypertension, insomnia, irritable bowel syndrome (IBS), mood swings, muscular tension, myalgia (muscle aches), neck pain, osteoarthritis, peptic ulcers, pinched nerves, poor posture, RSI, sciatica, snoring, sports injuries, stress, tennis elbow, tension, ulcers, varicose veins, wheezing and whiplash. It also helps breathing and voice control for singers, dancers, public speakers and actors.

How to find a teacher

It is essential to find a reputable teacher who has undergone at least 1,600 hours of training and has a certificate from a certified Alexander training school. If in any doubt about whom to go to, contact one of the national organizations listed in Part IV for a register of qualified teachers.

What to expect

Although a few Alexander teachers may provide group sessions, most of which will be introductory, the main teaching needs to be with one pupil only at a time. At the first session brief notes may be taken of your medical condition. You will be asked to wear loose garments and remain fully clothed throughout. To start with you will probably be asked to walk around, sit and stand up so that the teacher can watch how you use your body. Teachers are specially trained to observe and re-educate an individual's 'Use', which is Alexander's term for the way an organism works. Your teacher will have a thorough understanding and experience of change in his or her own manner of Use in using the technique every day.

The emotional and physical demands we undergo can become fixed in the body as, for instance, chronic muscular habits of muscular tension that cause the head, neck and back to be out of alignment. This in turn may cause rounded shoulders, a bowed head, arched back and back pain, with strain on the heart, lungs and digestive system. Even simple activities, such as reading a book, involve the use of many muscles, and there are very many instances of misplaced muscular activity. Teachers use gentle guidance with the hands to help unravel the distortions and at the same time encourage the natural reflexes (that is, what we are born with) to start working again.

You are taught to become aware of your habitual and unconscious reactions to situations, to 'inhibit' or stop those habits that create tension and to 'direct' yourself in a more poised, co-ordinated and 'free' manner. This will mean you have to let go of the habits of a lifetime. While you sit, stand or lie down, the teacher will gently guide and adjust your body with the hands. You will almost certainly react with old habits, may resist the changes or try to move your body in your familiar way. You will be taught how to inhibit these reactions, so that you can experience using your body in another way, with more freedom and ease. You will be taken very slowly through an apparently simple movement such as standing. The teacher will guide you through the action, time and time again, helping you to inhibit reactions of muscle contraction, while you learn a new way of moving. At the same time you will listen to and act on the teacher's instructions, all the time learning how to give yourself a series of 'directions' so that you can begin to replicate these changes for yourself outside lessons. By constantly thinking about and practising what you have learnt you will learn to use your body more freely, with minimum effort and maximum efficiency. Once you learn to let the muscles work in a harmonious, balanced and more efficient manner, the resulting improved posture will benefit your breathing, circulation and digestive systems as well as relieving musculo-skeletal problems. It will also benefit you as a whole. It may change your perception of yourself and how you live your life.

The technique does not consist of a set of exercises, rather, it is a way of living your daily life. It is neither quick nor easy to learn and is a long-term process that involves a lot of commitment and self-examination. To benefit fully, it is suggested you undertake a course of at least 30 lessons of 30–45 minutes each. Ideally, you will have lessons twice a week for the first 10–12 lessons, and these will drop down to once a week thereafter. The aim is for you to be able to continue on your own throughout your daily activities. As our habits are so strong, they will tend to return or new habits of tension may develop. Therefore, most people will need and want to have more lessons at a later date, to help them keep in touch with the technique.

Self treatment

You can help yourself by observing yourself and other people and watching how we move and what we do to our bodies.

During the first session, your teacher will ask you to lie down with your back on the floor with knees bent and feet flat on the ground for 15–20 minutes a day. Lie with your eyes open in a state of relaxed awareness while you give yourself directions, as you have been taught. There should be a book or books under your head to avoid neck strains. This will help ease your body into a less contracted, more open and free state.

Limitations and dangers

Alexander teachers are not trained to diagnose disorders or infectious diseases, some of which may need treatment before it is appropriate to take Alexander Technique lessons. There are no dangers in using the technique so long as you have been taught by a fully qualified Alexander teacher. If your teacher is not properly qualified you may be taught incorrectly and this may result in muscle strain and additional tension.

Anthroposophical medicine

Definition and principles

With anthroposophical medicine there are thought to be four distinct aspects of being human: the physical, the etheric, the sentient or 'astral' body and the 'I', the ego or self. These four aspects need to be kept in equilibrium for an individual to function properly, together with the three systems: the physical nerve/sense/skin system, the liver/digestive organs/muscles system and the rhythmic system, which functions through the heart, lungs and circulatory and respiratory systems. The latter interpenetrates the other two systems and enables the body to function properly in balance. Illness implies an imbalance, but imbalances are seen to be inevitable and as something to be viewed positively.

Brief outline

Anthroposophical medicine is based on the work of Rudolf Steiner (1861–1925), an Austrian scientist and philosopher who believed in reincarnation. It is currently practised widely in Switzerland and Germany.

Conditions helped

Anthroposophical practitioners are medically qualified so they can be consulted about any problem. The therapy has been particularly useful in alleviating anxiety, asthma, problems associated with cancer, depression, fatigue and musculoskeletal problems.

How to find a therapist

It is essential to find fully qualified practitioners. Contact a national organization (see Part IV).

What to expect

You will be asked detailed questions about your medical history and lifestyle and will have a physical examination as well as, if necessary, blood tests and other investigations. A diagnosis will include an orthodox medical diagnosis and an assessment of the state of your rhythmic system outlined above. Treatment includes anthroposophical medicines, derived from mineral, plant and animal sources, a special diet, massage and hydrotherapy. You may also be asked to undertake anthroposophical movements known as eurythmy, or art or music therapies.

Self treatment

Self treatment is an essential part of anthroposophical medicine. You will be expected to take a positive and active role in your treatment which will mean changing your lifestyle.

Limitations and dangers

Anthroposophical treatments cannot be proved to be effective, but they are not harmful and may prove beneficial where a conventional cure cannot help.

Aromatherapy

Definition and principles

Aromatherapy is the therapeutic use of pure essential oils, the aromatic essences of which are believed to contain medicinal properties and natural healing powers that improve the balance of body and mind. The essences are extracted from large quantities of various parts of medicinal and aromatic plants, flowers and trees. Once absorbed through the skin, they work rapidly. They are diluted in vegetable oils such as almond, sunflower, wheatgerm or avocado oil, or alcohol, and may have calming, toning, regulating or stimulating effects.

Aromatherapy is a holistic therapy that can be provided in conjunction with conventional medicine and is used both to alleviate many symptoms of illness and promote well-being and good health. The therapy supports the body in its fight against disease and as essential oils act as a catalyst they can stimulate the body to heal itself.

Brief outline

Treatment with essential oils can be traced back about 5,000 years. The medicinal use of plant oils is recorded in the early Egyptian and Persian empires, as well as in early Chinese writings.

At the beginning of the twentieth century a French chemist, Professor René-Maurice Gattefossé, found that essential oils could affect the skin in various ways. He discovered the healing power of lavender oil by accident when he plunged his hand into a basin full of the substance after receiving a bad burn in a laboratory accident. After a short while his hand healed without a scar. Gattefossé was particularly interested in the use of oils for skin problems such as dermatitis. He recognized their value as anti-bacterial agents and their potential for treating infections and also perceived the psychotherapeutic benefits of scents.

Gattefossé's work was later augmented by Marguerite Maury, a French biochemist who worked for the Guerlain scent firm. She investigated the properties of essential oils in the 1940s and used the oils together with massage. Her way was to treat the whole person: mind, body and spirit. A French physician, Dr Jean Valnet, used a different approach to essential oils in the 1950s. They were taken orally by his patients and helped to alleviate the symptoms of a number of diseases, including cancer, tuberculosis and diabetes.

It is not yet understood exactly how aromatherapy works. It is, however, known that essential oils stimulate the sense of smell. This in turn affects a region of the brain known as the limbic system, the activity of which is connected with instinctive behaviour, strong emotions and hormone control, which is why essential oils can temporarily alter mood and release stress. Essential oils can be absorbed through the skin and into the bloodstream, where they have been found to have a physiological effect on the nearby body tissue.

Studies have shown that older people can benefit very greatly from treatment, as aromatherapy can help to alleviate sleeplessness, anxiety, depression and the pain of arthritis. It is often used to offset the side-effects of drugs, and with treatment the intake of painkillers and sedatives can often be reduced.

In France, aromatherapy is part of orthodox medical treatment. In the UK it is the fastest growing alternative therapy and within the National Health Service many nurses are enthusiastically incorporating aromatherapeutic massage into their practice.

Conditions helped

Aromatherapy has been known to alleviate many problems and has particularly benefited the following conditions: acne, alopecia, anaemia, anger, anorexia nervosa, anxiety, arthritis, back pain, bedwetting, blisters, bronchitis, bruises, bulimia nervosa, bursitis, candidiasis, catarrh, colds, colic, constipation, coughs, cramp, croup, cystitis, dandruff, depression, diarrhoea, fainting, feeling run down, flatulence, frozen shoulder, gallstones, headaches, heavy periods, hyperventilation, hysteria, impetigo, indigestion, insomnia, irritable bowel syndrome (IBS), laryngitis, menopausal problems, myalgic encephalomyelitis (ME), migraine, mood swings, muscle strain, neck pain, neuralgia, night sweats, pain, panic attacks, peptic ulcers, phobias, post-natal depression, pre-menstrual syndrome (PMS), scalds, seasonal affective disorder (SAD), shock and trauma, sinusitis, sports injuries, spots and pimples, stress, sweating, tennis elbow, tension, tiredness, travel sickness, vaginitis and warts.

Aromatherapy treatment is excellent when used to alleviate the anxiety, pain and stress suffered by cancer patients. It may also reduce the side-effects of chemotherapy.

Four examples of essential oils and the symptoms they relieve are given below.

- *Eucalyptus oil* is a decongestant and helps with respiratory problems such as bronchitis, catarrh and influenza.

- *Juniper oil* helps with urinary problems and rheumatic joints.
- *Lavender oil* is an antiseptic. It is used for burns, bites and wounds. It helps with anxiety, insomnia, menstrual problems, migraine and pain.
- *Peppermint oil* helps to relieve nausea and vomiting.

How to find a therapist

It is essential to receive treatment from a fully trained, qualified and reputable aromatherapist. Contact one of the national organizations listed in Part IV.

What to expect

If you visit a practitioner with a particular problem, the initial session may last for up to two hours. There will be a detailed discussion about, and examination of, your general health, symptoms, emotions, way of life, exercise taken, skin type and sleeping habits.

Once a diagnosis has been made the practitioner will select appropriate oils, taking into account both your symptoms and a holistic view of your health. You may be asked to help choose your favourites by using your sense of smell. Essential oils will be chosen by the practitioner according to your specific needs. Each oil has an affinity with various parts of the body and encourages cellular activity. Combined with the therapeutic effects of massage, the oils help to improve the circulation and to eliminate toxins. They often have a comforting and soothing effect on your body and mind.

Oils may be applied or added to compresses, tinctures, lotions, creams or ointments to be used at home. Additionally, the practitioner uses essential oils diluted in a vegetable oil base on your body, together with a massage. A full massage will last for over an hour. The massage techniques used aim to release tension and improve circulation.

After massage you may experience a range of different reactions. For example, you may feel sleepy or your muscles may ache. Or you may get a headache, feel enlivened or more relaxed.

Self treatment

There are many essential oils that can be bought over the counter from chemists or health shops. It is, however, safer to buy them from an experienced practitioner who will be more likely to guarantee their quality. It is important to use only pure essential oils free from additives and to follow instructions for their dilution. They should be kept in dark coloured glass containers and protected from heat and sunlight.

It is advisable to buy oils blended by a qualified aromatherapist and to go on an aromatherapy course to learn the basics of the therapy and how to use the oils before you treat yourself.

Limitations and dangers

Essential oils are powerful chemicals and if used to excess may prove dangerously toxic. The following points should be borne in mind.

- It is *essential* to receive advice from a fully trained, qualified and reputable aromatherapist before undergoing any treatment.
- Aromatherapy is unregulated in almost every country in the world and there are very many untrained and unqualified people practising this therapy. Make sure you find a reputable therapist through a national organization. See Part IV for details.
- If you are prone to nose bleeds, have asthma, diabetes, epilepsy, high blood pressure or a skin condition, consult an aromatherapist for treatment. Do not self treat.
- If you are currently taking drugs or remedies supplied by other alternative therapists, always consult an aromatherapist. Do not self treat.
- Essential oils should be used with care. Some are toxic in large doses and may irritate the skin. With the exception of lavender oil for treating burns, *never* use any undiluted essential oil on the skin. Some essential oils such as cinnamon bark may cause an allergic skin reaction. Never apply oils to damaged skin. Note that aromatherapy may exacerbate serious skin infections such as eczema or psoriasis.
- Only ever ingest an essential oil prescribed by a practitioner who is qualified to administer essential oils orally.
- Note that some oils can exacerbate existing health problems.

- If you are pregnant, have treatment from a qualified practitioner. Do not treat yourself. The following oils should always be avoided in pregnancy: basil, camphor, hyssop, juniper, parsley, pennyroyal, sage, tarragon and wintergreen.
- Keep the oils away from fire as they are highly flammable.
- Do not use phototoxic oils prior to exposure to sunlight. These oils, such as bergamot or lemon oil, may irritate the skin or cause discoloration if exposed to direct sunlight or ultra-violet light.
- Do not have aromatherapy if you have any condition that may be caused by a serious underlying disease or a serious infection.

Art therapy

Definition and principles

Art therapy is a method of self-exploration using art materials.

Brief outline

The therapy was first used in the 1940s to rehabilitate shell-shocked soldiers. It has alleviated many emotional and psychological disturbances, and is often used in prisons, psychiatric hospitals and in schools for children with special needs. Art therapy is used for those who are 'beyond words' and for those who find it hard, or who are unable, to express their emotions verbally.

Conditions helped

Art therapy is used for a wide range of problems, including addictions, anxiety, bereavement problems, eating disorders, emotional disorders, emotions experienced relating to terminal illness, learning difficulties and low self-esteem. It is for those who have suffered severe trauma such as rape or torture, and those with post-traumatic stress disorders.

How to find a therapist

Ask your doctor or contact a national organization (see Part IV). In the UK you will be referred to an art therapist by your GP.

What to expect

You will be given art materials such as charcoal, clay, crayons, paints and plasticine, together with cardboard, old newspapers and paper. What you do with them is up to you. Your work will not be interpreted directly but you will be helped to understand what you have done and why. You may feel deep emotions such as rage and hatred and may perhaps relive a past trauma. A fully trained and experienced practitioner will help you to express these feelings safely. You will be helped to overcome a fear of self-expression and to gain confidence and self-esteem.

Weekly sessions last for up to one-and-a-half hours, either on a one-to-one basis or as part of a group.

Self treatment

Use art materials to relax and to allow problems to surface that need examining. Let yourself go. Work as quickly as you can so that you have no time to think or criticize what you are doing. Draw, paint or model the first things that come into your head. Afterwards, write down what you are thinking and feeling.

Limitations and dangers

You may find that surprisingly deep emotions and memories of long-buried painful experiences begin to emerge. Find a therapist whom you like and trust and who you feel can help you cope with these emotions. If you are treating yourself it is best to have someone nearby who can comfort you if necessary.

Autogenic training

Definition and principles

Autogenic therapy is based on the theory that the way we live creates imbalances and causes disease. Deep relaxation exercises help to rebalance these natural processes, control voluntary muscles and boost immune systems. Autogenic means 'generated from within'. The technique mobilizes our innate systems for healing and recuperation.

Brief outline

The therapy was developed by Dr Johannes Schultz, a German neurologist and hypnotherapist, in the 1920s. It has been used with great success in hospitals to help control mild hypertension and pain.

Conditions helped

The therapy is used primarily to promote good health and prevent disease. It also helps to alleviate addictions such as smoking, and curtail behavioural problems such as bedwetting, depression, panic attacks and stuttering. It may relieve tension and stress, reduce high blood pressure and is thought to be effective in alleviating Reynaud's disease. It has also been used to alleviate insomnia, asthma, irritable bowel syndrome (IBS) and migraine.

How to find a therapist

There are many orthodox practitioners who will recommend a reputable therapist. Otherwise contact one of the national organizations in Part IV for details.

What to expect

You will probably be taught in a group in weekly sessions lasting up to one-and-a-half hours for about ten weeks. Initially there is a medical check and psychological assessment, and you will be asked to fill in a comprehensive form listing your medical history. There are six basic exercises taught in sequence for which you lie down or sit and silently repeat phrases aimed to induce deep relaxation and peace. The first concentrates thoughts on the heaviness of certain limbs; the second on warmth in the limbs; the third focuses on the heartbeat; the fourth on an awareness of breathing; the fifth on the feeling of warmth in the abdomen; the sixth on the coolness of the forehead. You should keep a diary, note problems and compare notes with others. Self treatment is essential, and you will start to practise deep relaxation techniques after your first session. Once you have mastered the basic training you may want to learn more advanced techniques.

Limitations and dangers

Autogenic therapy is not recommended for anyone suffering a serious condition such as heart disease or glaucoma, diabetes or epilepsy, or for those with a serious psychiatric illness such as schizophrenia.

Autosuggestion

Definition and principles

Autosuggestion can be described as self-induced meditative hypnosis. A major principle is that the mind and body interact with each other.

Brief outline

The techniques of autosuggestion were devised in the late nineteenth century by Emile Coué, a French pharmacist. He found an individual's negative conscious thoughts could be eliminated by constantly repeating positive words or phrases and claimed such a positive mantra released the healing powers of the mind and body. Coué was convinced people could 'will' their recovery from illness by imagining themselves healed. His ideas have been incorporated into therapies such as visualization (see p. 139) and autogenic training (see above).

Conditions helped

Autosuggestion helps to alleviate and sometimes clear addictions, allergies, asthma, bronchitis, depression, pain, panic attacks, phobias, shock, stress and tension. It can foster self-confidence and positive attitudes.

How to find a therapist

It is important to learn autosuggestion techniques from a fully qualified hypnotherapist. Contact a national hypnotherapy organization (see Part IV) for further information.

Self treatment

Before you start, be clear about what you want to achieve. Think about what might be 'blocking' you, that is, preventing you from achieving. Lie or sit on a comfortable bed or chair, making sure nothing will distract you. Relax and try to release tension in your body. Empty your mind of extraneous thoughts. To achieve this, imagine a peaceful place where you feel happy: walking in the sun in a meadow or lying in the shade near a lake. Make a statement out loud about what you want, using positive words or phrases. Repeat this up to 20 times. Then, when you are ready, bring yourself out of the hypnotic state by gently letting go of the image you have created. You should practise autosuggestion regularly, twice a day, to achieve any benefit.

Limitations and dangers

Autosuggestion is unsuitable for anyone who has a serious unresolved conflict or who is suffering from a psychotic illness.

Ayurveda

Definitions and principles

The word 'Ayurveda' may be translated as 'life knowledge' or the 'science of life'. Its essence is balance. It is an ancient holistic system that places equal emphasis on treating the body, emotions, mind and spirit, and has been described as a complete guide to health, well-being and spiritual energy.

Treatment is based on realigning *prana*, the internal energy to promote health. Practitioners consider disease is created by an imbalance of the three humours or *doshas*, that is, the Vata, Pitta and Kapha. Vata can be correlated to the physical and mental activities ascribed to the nervous systems by modern physiology. The entire chemical process operating in your body can be attributed to Pitta, and the aspects of metabolism involved in constructing the physical body to Kapha. Ayurvedic treatments aim to rebalance the imbalance between these doshas. To find out more about the principles of the Ayurvedic system of holistic medicine, the underlying philosophy and methods of treatment, it is suggested you read some books on the subject such as *Ayurveda: Life, Health and Longevity*, by Robert Svoboda, *Ayurveda: The Ancient Indian Healing Art*, by Scott Gerson, or *The Complete Illustrated Guide to Ayurveda* by Gopi Warrier and Deepika Gunawant (see Further Reading for more information).

Brief outline

Ayurvedic medicine originated in the ancient Hindu civilization about 5,000 years ago. It was and still is the traditional medicine in India. During the nineteenth century, after the British annexed India, it fell into disrepute and Indian medical practitioners tended to follow the then Western medical orthodoxies. Once India gained independence in 1947, however, there was a strong move to return to ancient traditional practices. An Act in 1970 established a Central Council for Ayurveda to ensure proper training and to set up a register of established and qualified practitioners. This earned the practice a respectable reputation and now over 75 per cent of Ayurvedic practitioners are registered in India.

Conditions helped

Ayurveda offers treatment for almost all known ailments. Particular success has been achieved in the treatment of anorexia, anxiety, arthritis, asthma, backache, bruises, bulimia, burns, bursitis, candidiasis, catarrh, colds, colic, colitis, constipation, cystitis, diarrhoea, eczema, feeling run down, frozen shoulder, gout, haemorrhoids (piles), headaches, healing of wounds, high cholesterol levels, hyperactivity, indigestion, insomnia, irritable bowel syndrome (IBS), kidney stones, Ménière's disease, menopausal symptoms, metabolic problems, migraine, mouth ulcers, nappy rash, nausea, neuralgia, obesity, osteoarthritis, pre-menstrual syndrome (PMS), psoriasis, rheumatoid arthritis, sinusitis, skin rashes, sore throats, sprains, stress, teething, tinnitus, ulcers, water retention and worms.

How to find a therapist

It is essential to find a fully qualified and experienced practitioner. Consult only physicians with a BAMS degree (Bachelor of Ayurvedic Medicines and Surgery). Ayurvedic training is long and gruelling (six years) and there are only a limited number of practitioners in Western countries. Beware of charlatans. Contact an approved national organization (see Part IV) for information about bona fide practitioners.

What to expect

At the initial session, a very thorough investigation is made into your lifestyle and medical history. You will be asked about your present problem, current medication, lifestyle and the history of your family. You will be given a physical examination, and your skin, eyes, nails, tongue and pulse will be examined. Your physical and mental state will be taken into account to aid diagnosis before any treatment begins. Diagnosis and treatment take into account not only symptoms of ill health and diet but also external factors such as lifestyle, time of year and weather.

You may be asked to undergo a detoxification process that may take the form of an enema, laxative or washing out of the nasal passages. Your practitioner will make up a remedy, which may be prepared mostly from plants, and sometimes from minerals, sea shells, animal substances or metals, in the form of decoctions, powder or tincture, to suit your individual requirements. Treatment is a long-term process, and getting the right balance of doshas may take weeks or months. You may be recommended to undertake yoga (see p. 141), meditation (see p. 102), breathing exercises (see pp. 56–7) or to change your diet. Fasting is sometimes recommended.

Self treatment

Self treatment is not recommended. There are a number of Ayurvedic remedies available that may be bought over the counter which can be extremely useful when used appropriately, but only after consultation with an Ayurvedic doctor.

Limitations and dangers

Ayurveda is not helpful in medical emergencies or in acute life-threatening conditions, or where major surgical interventions are required.

There are very few orthodox practitioners who understand or accept Ayurvedic medicine as it is based on principles that are for the most part alien to allopathic medicine.

Bates method for better eyesight

Definition and principles

Practitioners of the Bates method for better eyesight claim to improve sight without the use of lenses or surgery and restore the natural habits of seeing that are lost through strain, tension and misuse of the eyes.

Brief outline

The method is alternative to orthodox medicine and originated with Dr William Bates (1865–1931), an American ophthalmologist. According to Bates, we use eye muscles that are finely balanced and easily disturbed by nervous stress and emotional pressure so that errors of refraction occur. We are led to believe eyesight can only deteriorate but this is not the case. Extremes of emotion, such as grief and rage, worsen eyesight and if these emotions are sustained changes may be permanent. Bates believed that lenses do not 'correct' eyesight but accelerate its deterioration. He developed a system of re-training by relaxation and specific exercises for eye muscles to correct bad habits and vision defects, some of which are described below.

Conditions helped

The Bates method helps all conditions for which glasses or contact lenses are prescribed, for example, myopia (short sight), hypermetropia (long sight), squints and astigmatism.

How to find a therapist

Contact a national organization (see Part IV).

What to expect

Over a period of up to ten weekly sessions, you learn to relax and focus your mind and eyes while seeing. To rest the eyes, close them and think about something agreeable. Or close and cover the eyes with the palms of both hands to exclude all light. This is called palming. To improve focusing, hold a pencil in each hand, one at arm's length and the other about 15 cm (6 in) in front of you. Focus first on one, blink, then focus on the other (the pencil on which you are not focusing will appear double). Another exercise involves swinging the head and body gently to and fro, with the eyes focused in the distance but moving with the head.

Self treatment

Self treatment is essential. Because you are performing a number of exercises at frequent intervals, you will have to organize your daily routine very carefully.

Limitations and dangers

There are some eye conditions, such as cataracts or glaucoma, that cannot be helped. Never perform the exercises while wearing glasses or contact lenses. Note that orthodox practitioners do not consider the Bates method to be a substitute for either lenses or surgery.

Bioenergetics

Definition and principles

Bioenergetics works to integrate bodily sensation, emotional expression, intellectual understanding and the symbolic and spiritual meaning of our lives.

Brief outline

The therapy was developed by Dr Alexander Lowen in the USA during the 1950s. He thought that negative attitudes and emotions affect body language, that is, the way we sit, move, stand and even breathe, and that we develop 'character armour' as a protection against psychological pain and suffering. Emotional states such as fear, embarrassment and anger are reflected in tense muscles shown in posture and stance. By working on the body, feelings expressed can be released to liberate both body and mind.

In the USA the therapy is known as Bioenergetic Analysis.

Conditions helped

Practitioners claim to alleviate and sometimes effect a disappearance of the following problems: asthma, fatigue, headaches, irritable bowel syndrome (IBS), peptic ulcers and wheezing. Bioenergetics helps people gain awareness of their bodies and enables those who suffer from a poor self-image to develop a positive attitude to themselves. It thus might be useful in helping conditions related to low self-esteem such as depression, eating disorders and addictions.

How to find a therapist

Contact a national organization (see Part IV).

What to expect

Following a thorough assessment, your practitioner may recommend one-to-one therapy, or group sessions. Exercises to unlock the character armouring which enable the body to regain its ability to function freely focus on three main areas.

- *Breathing*: irregularities in breathing patterns, such as hyperventilation, may be caused by chronic muscular tensions owing to emotional suffering.
- *Character structure*: there are five major character structures in bioenergetics. Each individual will display elements of more than one type.
- *Grounding*: practitioners believe it is through our legs and feet that we manage to keep in contact with reality. You learn to connect with the ground so that you can both literally and metaphorically 'stand on your own two feet'.

Limitations and dangers

Bioenergetics can arouse very deep emotions. It is vital you are with a qualified and experienced practitioner who can deal creatively with the emotions expressed.

Biofeedback training

Definition and principles

Biofeedback training has been defined as 'a procedure that allows us to tune in to our bodily functions and, eventually, to control them'. It is a therapeutic technique that uses instruments to measure, amplify and provide continuous feedback on specific autonomic, that is, involuntary, bodily responses. It is based on the principle that these bodily responses can be regulated and then used to help alleviate certain conditions and maintain health and well-being.

Brief outline

There have been many successful trials and over 2,500 papers written about the subject. Almost all the papers strongly indicate, in ways that are not yet understood, that the therapy works to alleviate many problems. In the main, orthodox practitioners accept that the effects the instruments measure are accurate, and many now use biofeedback training in conjunction with allopathic medicine.

In the early 1930s scientists began to develop electronic devices to detect autonomic responses. Most of the instruments (see below) now used in biofeedback were originally designed for use in scientific and medical research in the 1950s and 1960s. With the rapid development of more sophisticated electronic equipment there was increasing interest in the subject. It was at this time that Dr Joe Kamiya was monitoring individuals' alpha wave activity in the brain, using electroencephalograph (EEG) machines. Dr Kamiya found that most of his subjects were able either to 'turn on' or consciously suppress alpha waves, indicating that EEG activity could be altered deliberately by means of feedback of EEG information to the subject. Thirty years later, it is known that all parts of the brain are intrinsically responsive to information, and that the brain responds to information about itself, including information provided externally by biofeedback. The impact of biofeedback training is reflected very strongly in severe cerebral illnesses such as epilepsy, traumatic brain injury, cerebral palsy and senile dementia, as well as irrational violence, criminal behaviour and addictive behaviour.

Today, the EEG is only one of a number of biofeedback devices (which do not affect the body in any way but simply provide information). For example, an electrocardiograph (ECG) monitors heart rate, while an electromyograph (EMG) measures muscular activity, tension and blood pressure and an electrical skin resistance meter measures skin temperature.

There have been many problems that scientific trials have shown to have been helped by biofeedback training. For instance, in 1991 a trial using biofeedback training showed that high blood pressure and tachycardia (abnormally rapid heart rate) were much reduced. Another trial in 1992 demonstrated the beneficial effect biofeedback had on tension headaches, while in the same year a US government report found that patients could successfully control incontinence using the technique. Another US study in 1996 showed that using biofeedback together with autogenic training helped to control involuntary muscle spasms after brain damage. It has also been found that using biofeedback training to lower forehead temperature has proved very effective in treating migraines and Raynaud's disease.

Conditions helped

The long list of conditions alleviated and in many cases eventually eliminated by biofeedback training include the following: addictions, anxiety, backache, Bell's palsy, breathing disorders, Carpal tunnel syndrome, depression, epilepsy, faecal incontinence, feeling run down, headaches, high blood pressure, hyperventilation, insomnia, irritable bowel syndrome (IBS), Ménière's disease, menopausal problems, menstrual cramps, migraines, muscle disorders, multiple sclerosis, myalgic encephalomyelitis (ME), neck pain, neuralgia, palpitations, postoperative pain, post-traumatic stress disorder, pre-menstrual syndrome (PMS), Raynaud's disease, stress, stroke, tinnitus, urinary incontinence and vertigo.

Biofeedback training can also be a very useful adjunct to bioenergetics (see p. 49), the Alexander Technique (see p. 31), autogenic training (see p. 42), meditation (see p. 102) and breathing and relaxation techniques (see p. 55), or where the patient is unable or unwilling to take oral treatments.

How to find a therapist

Contact one of the national organizations listed in Part IV for a qualified practitioner.

What to expect

Electrodes emanating from a biofeedback device are attached to your skin to provide information about your physiological responses, for example, blood pressure or pulse and sweat on the skin. These are involuntary processes controlled by the autonomic nervous system. Signals such as electronic bleeps, flashes, clicks or waves on a screen feed back physiological information to both you and your practitioner.

You first learn how to develop a state of relaxed awareness. To enable you to do this the practitioner will teach you one of a number of different techniques. For instance, you may be asked to think specific thoughts or feel specific emotions, control your rate of breathing, use visualization or progressive muscular relaxation techniques or meditate to achieve the desired result. Once you have learnt to enter a state of relaxed awareness, with the help of the practitioner you then learn to change the electronic signals. For example, you may learn to alter the width of a wave on the screen, the number of clicks heard per minute or the tone or pitch of a sound. In this way, you acquire the skill consciously to alter bodily functions that are involuntary, such as heart beat, peristaltic (intestinal) movements or sweating. You do this in order to alleviate the problem that has been diagnosed which may be, for example, high blood pressure, stress, pain or an addiction. Initially you may find it difficult to learn the techniques required and you may need ten or more sessions. Also, you will need regular follow-up to monitor your biofeedback ability.

Self treatment

Once you learn to achieve the state of mind required, you can practise biofeedback techniques anywhere, without using electrodes or machines. Unfortunately, though, it has been found that without mechanical feedback, biofeedback skills are often lost. It is not like riding a bicycle where once learnt the skill is remembered for ever. Much of the machinery involved is fairly simple to use, however, and provided you can afford to buy the necessary equipment required to control your particular problems, you can use it at home.

Limitations and dangers

Biofeedback is not suitable for any serious infection or conditions caused by serious underlying disease, except hypertension. Although there may be metabolic changes as a result of treatment, it is extremely important to note that you should never change the dosage of any prescribed medication without first consulting a doctor.

Biorhythms

Definitions and principles

The theory of biorhythms suggests an individual's life is influenced by physical, emotional and intellectual cycles.

Brief outline

During the 1900s, two people independently concluded that a unique 23-day cycle governing physical health operated for each individual. This influences strength, stamina, sex-drive, confidence, co-ordination and immunity to and recovery from illness. It runs concurrently with a 28-day cycle governing emotional health that influences nervous reactions, mood and creativity. Later, another cycle of 33 days was deemed to govern intellectual capacity. This influences decision-making, memory and concentration. These cycles operate from birth.

Conditions helped

Today, biorhythm charts are used to help individuals take precautions at times of physical and emotional illness. They also pinpoint days when they can best perform. Charts are useful for planning operations, marriages, moving house and business ventures, anything that depends both on success and avoiding risk. They can help older people plan ahead, to be active on 'good' days and to conserve energy on 'bad' ones.

How to obtain further information

You can obtain a computer printout of up to a year's biorhythmic forecasts from specialist agencies. Contact a 'general' national organization (see Part IV) for more information.

What to expect

When charted in months, the cycles form waves across a central horizontal line, known as the 'caution' line. The cycles coincide only rarely because they vary in length. When a cycle peaks an individual will be positive and active in that particular sphere. When it is in a trough, however, the individual will be negative and passive. Critical days occur when the cycles cross the caution line. When two or (very rarely) all three cycles intersect at this point the individual is said to be very vulnerable.

Self treatment

You can work out your own biorhythm chart using a biorhythmic calculator or special computer program.

Limitations and dangers

There is no scientific evidence for biorhythms. They will not cure you of any disease, and they cannot accurately predict accidents or crises.

Breathing and relaxation

Definition and principles

Both orthodox and alternative practitioners acknowledge that breathing and relaxing properly are essential for physical and mental well-being and for preventing ill health. Breathing forms a bridge between the body and mind as it can be consciously controlled, even though it is directed by the autonomic nervous system. Once breathing techniques have been mastered, learning to relax becomes very much easier.

Breathing and relaxation techniques form the basis of many alternative therapies.

Brief outline

Breathing and relaxation have been the basis of many traditional systems of medicine, including yoga and Traditional Chinese Medicine (TCM), where techniques for breathing efficiently and maintaining the interaction with the body and mind to cope with anxiety and stress, and to control *Qi* (life force), have been used for thousands of years.

In the 1960s, research into transcendental meditation found that sitting in a quiet environment and focusing the mind could reverse the effects of stress. A recent UK study has found that children with asthma reported a significant reduction in their problems by using breathing and relaxing techniques, while another recent study in the USA found that eight out of ten children with persistent headaches who had relaxation training found their condition improved. An increasing number of hospitals and health centres in the West are using breathing and relaxation techniques to help to calm patients and relieve anxiety and stress both before and after operations.

Conditions helped

Learning to breathe properly and relax help to alleviate many conditions. The techniques used are particularly important for the following conditions: agoraphobia, anxiety, asthma, childbirth, claustrophobia, dental treatment, depression, eczema, endometriosis, fatigue, hyperactivity, hysteria, insomnia, irritable bowel syndrome (IBS), high blood pressure, panic attacks, peptic ulcers, pre-menstrual syndrome (PMS), pain relief, repetitive strain injury (RSI), stammering and stuttering, stress and tension.

How to find a therapist

There are very few therapists who practise only breathing and relaxation techniques. Contact a national organization of a therapy that lays emphasis on breathing and relaxation, for example, the Alexander Technique, meditation, qigong, visualization, t'ai chi or yoga (see Part IV for addresses).

What to expect

If you visit a practitioner you will be asked about your medical history and anything that may be causing stress and anxiety. You will be asked to sit in a chair, lie on a couch or on a mat on the floor. The practitioner will talk you through various breathing and relaxation techniques and may suggest some exercises for you to do at home. The first session will probably last for an hour and second and subsequent sessions for slightly less. Most techniques can be learnt in about five sessions.

Self treatment

Breathing and relaxation exercises are easy to learn and they are essential if you want to keep fit or to help with healing. It is best to consult a practitioner to ensure you learn the techniques correctly, otherwise you will not benefit.

Before going to a therapist you can find out how you breathe and whether there is anything you can do to improve your breathing. There are two basic types of breathing: chest and abdominal. Chest breathing occurs when we physically exert ourselves, or feel fear, anxiety or anger: in short, when we need to take flight or fight and tense ourselves. Abdominal breathing that promotes relaxation should occur for most of the time, when we are relaxed. Unfortunately, those of us who live with permanent anxiety, tension and stress seem to have forgotten how to breathe abdominally, and this may have to be consciously relearned.

First, find a place where you will not be interrupted. Remove your shoes and loosen any tight clothing. Lie on a firm but comfortable surface (not a bed), and support your head with a pillow. To find out about chest breathing, place your hands on your upper chest (for women, above the breasts) and slowly breathe in and out through your mouth, making sure you use your chest muscles. Your hands should rise with each breath you take in and fall with each breath expelled. With chest breathing, breathing is fast and shallow. The rib muscles contract and this forces the chest to

THE THERAPIES

expand upwards and outwards with air being drawn quickly into the upper chest. If chest breathing continues for too long it may become a regular breathing habit.

Once you are aware of what chest breathing means you can progress to abdominal breathing. This time lie down and place one hand on the upper chest as before, and the other hand on the abdomen. Breathe in and out slowly as before but this time through the nose. Try to breathe so that only the lower hand, the one on the abdomen, moves. If you are tense you will find this difficult to do, if not impossible. Once you have managed to do this, place both hands on the abdomen and breathe in slowly through the nose. The abdomen should rise and the diaphragm move down, while the chest should be nearly still. Hold your breath for five seconds and slowly breathe out through the nose. Repeat this five times. Try to relax. Concentrate on the breathing rather than any stray thoughts that might enter your head. If you feel dizzy or faint, stop at once: you are putting far too much effort into what should be a slow, gentle and relaxed exercise. Good abdominal breathing is the basis of relaxation as it ensures there is a balance of oxygen and carbon monoxide in the bloodstream. It not only helps the body and mind to release physical and mental tension but also helps to alleviate quick and shallow breathing induced by stress.

Limitations and dangers

Some of the techniques used may release long-held pent-up emotions such as anger and grief, so it is important that if you are not with a practitioner when you do your breathing exercises you are with someone who can support you. If this is not possible, allow as much time as you need to experience these strong feelings and then slowly let them go.

Buteyko method

Definition and principles

The Buteyko method is based on the premise that dysfunctional breathing results in some manifestation of disease. When breathing is normalized many of the problems associated with disease may be alleviated and eventually eliminated.

Brief outline

The therapy is based on the work of a Russian scientist, Professor K P Buteyko who, after a great deal of research in Russia earlier in the twentieth century, discovered a connection between dysfunctional breathing and many diseases. The drug-free therapy retrains breathing patterns to increase oxygenation of blood and tissues. People are taught to breathe properly using their abdominal muscles and shallow breathing.

Although the therapy is very new and as yet not well known in the West there has already been some research conducted in Australia in 1994 that has shown that asthma may be greatly alleviated with the use of this method.

Conditions helped

Practitioners claim that the following problems have been alleviated and in some cases eliminated with the use of the Buteyko method: allergies, asthma, breathlessness, bronchitis, chronic fatigue, coughing, hayfever, high blood pressure and wheezing. The method may also help to increase energy levels and with losing weight.

How to find a therapist

Contact a 'general' national organization at the beginning of Part IV for further information.

What to expect

You will undergo training to correct any breathing irregularities and to recondition the breathing mechanism. You will learn some breathing exercises over a number of sessions and will be expected to practise these on your own.

Limitations and dangers

It is essential to be taught the Buteyko method by a reputable and fully qualified practitioner. If you do not learn the techniques properly you will almost certainly not gain any benefit and may well harm yourself.

Chiropractic

Definition and principles

The word 'chiropractic' is formed from two Greek words *kheir*, meaning hand, and *praktikos*, to use, meaning 'done by hand'. Chiropractors diagnose by feeling, which they term 'palpation', and treat disorders of the spine, joints and muscles by manual adjustment, quite often with the help of X-rays. They aim to improve function, relieve pain and increase mobility. Their main focus is on the spinal vertebrae but they also work on the muscles, ligaments, joints, bones and tendons. They claim that the manipulative process can have a positive effect on the nervous system and can even relieve conditions such as asthma and IBS that are not musculo-skeletal, as well as ones that are. Drugs and surgery are never used because practitioners, like most adherents of alternative therapies, believe in the vital force or homeostasis. They claim that when body systems are in harmony, the body can heal itself from within.

Brief outline

Spinal manipulation dates back at least 2,000 years. The ancient Greeks, Egyptians, Chinese, Hindus and Babylonians are known to have used manipulation to treat a range of health problems.

A North American, Daniel David Palmer (1845–1913), was the founder of modern chiropractic. He based his ideas on the beliefs of Hippocrates who stated the spine should be scrutinized for the basic cause of disease. Palmer knew that the spine protects the spinal cord and nerves emanating from the spine. He considered that if any section were to be disturbed, however slightly, this would cause an interference with some of the nerve impulses travelling through the spinal cord. This interference would prevent what he called the 'innate intelligence', that is, the vital force (*prana* or *Qi*) from passing through the body. Palmer concluded that if the parts of the spine that had been disturbed were to be readjusted, this would once more allow nerve impulses to travel freely.

Chiropractic treatment first became available in the USA at the end of the nineteenth century and in Europe a little before the First World War. Initially there was great opposition to the practice from orthodox practitioners. Bartlett J Palmer, the son of D D Palmer who followed in his father's footsteps and continued to develop chiropractic, was described as 'the most dangerous man in Iowa out of a prison cell'. At the end of the twentieth century, however, chiropractic has achieved worldwide respectability and legislation relating to its practice exists in nearly 20 countries, including Australia, Canada, New Zealand, the UK and the USA. It is now the most widely used, and probably the most respected, alternative therapy with around 60,000 practitioners worldwide.

Chiropractic's main focus has always been on the relationship between the impaired movement of spinal vertebrae and the central nervous system, and the effect this has on health. Practitioners claim that most problems relating to the spine stem from misalignments, maladjustments and excessive strain placed on joints. They call these problems 'subluxations', that is, small displacements. Subluxations may be caused by inherited skeletal distortions, poor posture, previous injuries, strains or stresses. Previous injuries or poor posture, strains or stresses resulting from physical or, more likely, emotional stress or poor self-image can interfere with, and impinge on, the nerves that emanate between the vertebrae, resulting in nerve dysfunction. The spine may have become misaligned and health impaired. There are many types of adjustment, the word chiropractors prefer to manipulation, that can be applied to joints, muscles and bodily tissues. The art of chiropractic is knowing how, when and where to perform these adjustments so that normal healthy mechanical function of the spine is restored. The chiropractor has to find out not only what has gone wrong but why, so that advice can be given about how to reduce or eliminate pain and correct bad habits.

There are variants on the traditional form of chiropractic. For example, McTimoney chiropractic adjusts individual bones using a fast, dextrous technique known as the toggle-torque-recoil. This makes the treatment particularly gentle to receive and it is very suitable for treating animals. McTimoney-Corley chiropractors practise a technique that uses only the fingertips, known as the 'reflex coil' adjustment, which is a light method of vertebral adjustment.

Around 80 per cent of the world's population suffer back problems at some point during their lives. In spite of improvements in diagnostic techniques, disability from back pain, particularly lower back pain, appears to be getting much worse. This is probably partly owing to how we use our bodies when we work with new technology, for example, the way we sit when working on computers. It may, however, also be the result

THE THERAPIES

of the way orthodox practitioners have traditionally treated back pain, that is, with ample and sometimes prolonged bed rest. This passive treatment seems to be proving less effective than active manipulative treatment such as chiropractic, which is able to treat most common musculo-skeletal problems, including arthritic and rheumatic conditions.

A study conducted under the auspices of the British Medical Research Council and published in the *British Medical Journal* in 1990 showed that patients with acute or chronic lower back pain of mechanical origin obtained excellent results with chiropractic treatment. It was significantly more effective than hospital outpatient treatment or physiotherapy. There was a follow-up study in 1995 with chiropractic showing a significant improvement over hospital outpatient treatment.

Conditions helped

Practitioners and patients claim the following conditions are alleviated and sometimes eliminated by chiropractic: anxiety, arm pains, asthma, back pain, catarrh, chest pain, constipation, digestive disorders, dislocations, dizziness, frozen shoulder, hay fever, headaches, heartburn, hip problems, indigestion, irritable bowel syndrome (IBS), joint pains, knee problems, lumbago (lower back pain), migraine, muscle and postural problems, neck pains, neuralgia, neurological disorders, numbness, painful periods, pins and needles, postural problems associated with pregnancy, rheumatism, sciatica, shoulder pains, slipped disc, sports injuries, strains, tinnitus and vertigo.

How to find a therapist

Orthodox practitioners are increasingly referring patients to chiropractors, so you might consider asking your doctor for a referral to a reputable practitioner. If, however, this is not possible, contact one of the national organizations listed in Part IV.

What to expect

At the first session your practitioner will take detailed notes of your medical history and will concentrate on your lifestyle. You may be advised to change your diet and to take more rest and/or exercise. Detailed diagnostic tests will then be carried out and the function of the spinal column, joints and muscles will be examined very carefully. The practitioner will examine you, feeling for areas of muscle spasm, pain and tenderness to find out which joints are moving properly and which are not. X-rays are used if the chiropractor thinks they are necessary. Your posture will be examined and any signs of bone or muscle injury or disease will be noted. The chiropractor will then decide whether or not you are a suitable candidate for chiropractic treatment. If not, you will be advised to see a medical practitioner.

If, however, chiropractic is deemed to be suitable, you may be asked to strip to your underclothes. Treatment may mean you will stand, sit or lie on a special chiropractic couch. Your chiropractor may use his or her hands to adjust the joints of the spine using slight pressure and rapid thrusts on the vertebrae. The treatment is intended to stretch muscles, unlock joints and correct problems in parts of the body that originate from the spine. You may also receive massage of the muscles. This is to relieve muscle spasm and pain and also to prepare a joint for adjustment treatment.

Your chiropractor will treat what is known as a 'fixation', that is, a restriction of movement in a joint affecting other structures and tissues. He or she will adjust the spine, using only the hands, to restore a full range of movement and relax the muscles. In this way, inflammation and pain will be reduced. You may experience immediate relief from symptoms, though it is more likely that several treatments will be necessary before you get better. You may feel sore, stiff or ache a bit after treatment.

Self treatment

You cannot self-treat with chiropractic. Nevertheless, there are a series of simple but very important preventive exercises that have been devised for taking in between treatments. These ensure the treatment holds and help you to take control of your own recovery and body. They also help you to embrace a healthier lifestyle. The exercises will be outlined by the practitioner.

Limitations and dangers

Chiropractic is not suitable if you have any condition requiring surgery, suffer from bone malignancy, trapped nerves, if there is any inflammation or if there are any signs of infection or tumours in the spine. The therapy is also not advisable if you suffer from gout or osteoarthritic hips. There are, however, relatively few situations where chiropractic is unsuitable,

THE THERAPIES

though these may differ depending on the technique practised. McTimoney and McTimoney-Corley treatments, for example, are so gentle that patients with osteoporosis can be treated.

You must receive treatment from a qualified and registered chiropractor. If you are treated by someone who is not fully trained in the specialized techniques, this could cause you harm. Qualified chiropractors are trained to identify conditions that should not be treated and will refer you on to an appropriate practitioner or your doctor.

Colour therapy

Definition and principles

Modern colour therapy is rooted in psychology and parapsychology. Colour is seen to relate to the aura and chakras as well as to physical, emotional and mental states.

Brief outline

Human attitudes and behaviours are greatly influenced by colour. For instance, we equate purple with rage, red with anger, green with envy and silver with fluent speech ('silver tongued'). It is suggested that all colours used appropriately can counteract illness and enhance lifestyles. Colour therapists believe that an unbalanced body or mind lacks, or is overloaded by, particular colours and aim to create harmony by increasing or reducing these colours accordingly. Red, orange and yellow are perceived to be 'hot', while blue, indigo and violet are 'cold'. Green acts as a balancer.

Conditions helped

The therapy has successfully reduced obsessive-compulsive behaviour and has also helped schizophrenics and those suffering from depression, asthma, inflammatory and metabolic conditions.

How to find a therapist

Although it is easy to find practitioners in the USA, colour therapy is not as well known in other countries. There are very few organizations that cater solely for colour therapy. Contact a 'general' national organization in Part IV for a recommended therapist.

What to expect

At the first consultation the practitioner takes details of your medical history and lifestyle, particularly noting diet and colour preferences, and concentrates on your body language and aura, seeking psychic vibrations. You will be asked to eat foods, wear clothes, and live in rooms surrounded by certain colours. During sessions coloured light is beamed on to various parts of your anatomy. You will need about ten treatments.

Self treatment

Although you need guidance from an experienced practitioner, self help is a vital part of the healing process as you have to make substantial changes to your lifestyle.

Limitations and dangers

The therapy is quite safe but not recommended for serious illnesses, unless used as an adjunct to other therapies.

Crystal and gem therapies

Definition and principles

Although crystal and gem therapies are somewhat different in practice, both have the same core principles. Practitioners believe that crystals and gem stones have vibrational characteristics that help healing, and that by using them an individual's energies can be balanced and focused.

Brief outline

There has been a very long history of a belief in the healing power of gems and crystals, which used to be crushed and mixed with wine and drunk, or used as lotions for wounds and as antidotes for poison. Each stone had specific attributes, many of which are still recognized today. For example, a moonstone protected travellers and stimulated the mind, while an emerald helped strengthen eyesight and cured dysentery. Crystals that are used as microchips in computers, watches and radios, for example, may be programmed with healing energy.

Conditions for use

Specific conditions are not treated. Crystal and gem therapies are often used as adjuncts to other therapies: they enhance the process of healing in the treatment of any physical or emotional condition.

How to find a therapist

Always consult a registered practitioner who should have trained for a minimum of two years part-time (at least 100 hours of teaching and six months of home study).

What to expect

On your first visit you will be asked in detail about your lifestyle, diet and medical history. You will then be asked to sit or lie on a couch or on the floor, without undressing. You may have gems or crystals placed around you or on specific parts of your body, or they may be held, either by you or the practitioner, who will tap into their healing energy. You may be asked to visualize healing energy emanating through the stones and may be given a gem or crystal to wear, carry or be placed in a room in your home.

Limitations and dangers

There is no danger with either therapy but there have been no clinical trials to provide evidence for effectiveness of treatment.

Dance therapy

Definition and principles

Dance therapy uses movement to bypass the conscious mind and make contact with the unconscious inner emotional world. The aim is to bring up images that raise important emotional issues for the patient.

Brief outline

Modern dance therapy was developed by Rudolph Laban in the early twentieth century. He believed that dance could benefit an individual's mental condition and created new dance forms that enabled the mind and body to act in harmony.

Conditions helped

The dance therapist suggests movements that might give the patient a stronger sense of identity. Movement may also resolve disturbing issues that occurred before the patient learnt to speak. The therapy is used to improve posture and breath control, encourage relaxation, help concentration, develop playfulness and creativity, promote self-esteem and gain insight into emotional problems. It helps those who have been abused or traumatized; with physical and learning difficulties; suffering depression or anxiety; or those with psychotic or eating disorders and senile dementia. Dance therapy is often practised combined with physiotherapy or occupational therapy.

How to find a therapist

Contact a national organization (see Part IV). It is essential to find a practitioner who has trained for at least two years full-time.

What to expect

Dance therapy is practised either one-to-one or in groups. There is no set routine because so much depends on spontaneous expression, but usually there are three distinct stages. Sessions may begin with warm-ups to increase body awareness and ease joints. Music is then played with patients making movements to the music, or patients may make their own music together with spontaneous movements. The therapist watches the movements, or dances along with the patient, or mirrors the patient's actions. At the end of each session feelings that have been aroused are discussed. With a group, the therapist assesses the group dynamics and how participants relate to others while they move.

Limitations and dangers

Dance therapy is not good for those who suffer from arthritis, back problems or very high blood pressure.

Feldenkrais method

Definition and principles

The Feldenkrais method is an educational system that teaches people to move easily with minimum effort and maximum efficiency. This positively affects their entire physical, emotional and mental well-being.

Brief outline

The method was developed by a Russian-Israeli scientist, Dr Moshe Feldenkrais, who adapted both Eastern and Western body concepts to form a series of exercises. He concentrated on the body in motion. Movements are gentle with the focus on becoming more aware of and sensitive to how they are performed. It is *not* about achieving goals or doing better, but about moving and breathing with less strain and tension. You are taught a new awareness of crawling and walking, how each part of you, your head, eyes, pelvis, spine and limbs move in relation to each other, and how to become conscious of breathing while moving.

Conditions helped

The Feldenkrais method helps to improve balance and co-ordination and helps to alleviate back and neck pain, clumsiness, other musculoskeletal or neurological problems, and poor self-image. It improves digestion, sleep patterns, alertness and flexibility. It has been used to help accident victims.

How to find a therapist

Contact a Feldenkrais organization (see Part IV) for a fully qualified teacher who should have trained part-time for at least four years or 800 hours.

What to expect

There are two Feldenkrais techniques. A Functional Integration lesson is one-to-one and you will be shown new ways of moving. With lessons in Awareness Through Movement you will be in a group and led through a series of gentle movements. The exercises are centred around sitting and walking. The lessons are simple to start with and evolve into complicated techniques using guided imagery to imagine a new way of moving. These are repeated many times until you find them easy to do and become wholly aware of what you are doing.

Limitations and dangers

The Feldenkrais method is not recommended for anyone with a severe disability. The long-term effects of the treatment have not yet been studied.

Flotation therapy

Definition and principles

Flotation therapy is a method of isolating the mind and body from external stimuli to induce deep relaxation.

Brief outline

The therapy evolved in the 1970s through work by John C Lilly, an American doctor, psychoanalyst and neuro-physiologist in Washington DC. Initially, flotation tanks were known as sensory deprivation chambers and it was some time before the benefits of external stimuli deprivation were realized.

Conditions helped

Flotation therapy has helped with addictions, such as smoking, overeating or alcoholism. It has also helped to reduce aching muscles, anxiety, arthritis, back pain, depression, headaches, high blood pressure, insomnia, migraines, muscle fatigue, pain, stress and ulcers. In addition it has helped with problems associated with heart disease and multiple sclerosis. The sensation of being 'held' by the water in the tank is calming and reassuring and is thought to resemble inter-uterine life.

How to find a therapist

You must find a well-qualified practitioner. Contact one of the flotation organizations or one of the 'general' organizations listed in Part IV for further information.

What to expect

After taking a shower, you enter an enclosed tank about 2.5 m (8 ft) long, 1.25 m (4 ft) wide, filled with about 25 cm (10 in) water, to which have been added salts and minerals to ensure you float effortlessly. Ear plugs insulate against sound and also protect against the salts and minerals. You lie in near or total darkness and silence, with water kept at skin temperature around 93 degrees F (34 degrees C) for up to two-and-a-half hours. Both mind and body become very relaxed, and you may feel disembodied. After treatment you will probably have more control over your emotions and experience a sense of well-being, because floating stimulates the body's production of endorphins, natural substances produced by the body to relieve pain. It has been suggested that one hour of flotation therapy is the equivalent of six hours of sleep.

Limitations and dangers

The therapy is not recommended for those suffering any form of psychosis, severe depression or any type of phobia, particularly claustrophobia. Consult your doctor before treatment.

Flower remedies

Definition and principles

Flower remedies are taken from wild plants, bushes and trees. They are collected at auspicious times of the day and placed in crystal bowls filled with pure spring water. These are left in sunlight which is believed to 'potentize' the spring water with the 'essence' or 'auric pattern' of the plant. This liquid is then diluted many times to form the stock remedies sold in bottles.

Brief outline

For thousands of years healers have used flowers to help heal the sick. Dr Edward Bach, who created flower remedies in England during the early part of the twentieth century, had an intuitive knowledge of plants and made an in-depth study of personality types. He believed physical problems manifested as a result of dis-ease, a conflict of the emotions. Flower remedies, he claimed, harmonized the imbalances of the psyche.

Flower remedies have been developed using flowers from all over the world, particularly Australia, England, India, New Zealand, Scotland and various parts of the USA.

Conditions helped

Physical problems related to emotions and stress seem to respond to treatment. Flower remedies are particularly helpful in alleviating agoraphobia, amnesia, anxiety, claustrophobia, depression, fear and manic depressive disorders. They treat the whole person, rather than specific symptoms or ailments, and aim to harmonize mind, body and spirit. Dr Bach's rescue remedy has been claimed to have saved many lives following shock, haemorrhage and accidents.

How to find a therapist

Contact a national organization (see Part IV).

What to expect

Suitable remedies will be prepared and you will be told exactly what each remedy is for, how much to take, when it should be taken and what effects it will have. The length of treatment varies from weeks to many months. For example, it will be several months before an improvement is noticed when remedies are taken to work on deep-seated emotional problems.

Self treatment

An experienced practitioner will assess the required treatment, but you can make up your own remedies or buy them from reputable health stores.

Limitations and dangers

There are no dangers.

Healing

Definition and principles

Healers can restore people to health by channelling healing energy to activate the body which is thought to stimulate homeostasis, the self-healing balance mechanism. Faith is not necessary but an open mind is essential.

THE THERAPIES

Brief outline

Healing was practised in ancient Egypt and was recognized in Greece. Although there are many instances of healing in the Bible, Christianity tended to link healing powers to pagan religions. Between the fifteenth and seventeenth centuries 'psychics' and healers in Europe were persecuted and some 300,000 murdered. The rift between the material and the spirit (and the body and spirit) widened, as the mechanistic world view spread. Ill health was seen to be related only to the body, the mind was only occasionally considered and the spirit totally ignored.

In the twentieth century, however, healing once more became an accepted therapeutic practice, and in the UK it is now the most used unorthodox therapy. There are around 12,000 healers attached to reputable healing organizations and an estimated total of around 20,000. A doctor-healer network exists and the patients' charter introduced by the UK government in 1990 entitled patients in NHS hospitals to request the services of healers as complementary to orthodox treatment.

Much research has taken place on the efficacy of healing, including controlled trials.

Conditions helped

Healers treat all problems. Practitioners claim the following conditions have particularly benefited from treatment: anxiety, depression, headaches, heavy periods, migraine, neuralgia, post operative pain, PMS, phobias, panic attacks, post-traumatic stress disorders, stress and tension. Those suffering from the sadness and grief of bereavement have also benefited.

How to find a healer

Anyone can set up as a healer, so beware of charlatans – and particularly people who charge large fees. Note that in the UK most healers do not make a charge; they may accept donations according to a person's ability to pay. Some who work full-time, however, do charge a fee. You are advised not to rely on the advice of your friends or on advertisements but to contact a reputable organization that complies with mandatory regulations, including training, a probationary service and one that provides insurance cover.

What to expect

There are many ways in which healers operate. The following applies to contact healers. These think of themselves as channels of healing energies that work through them rather than come from them. There are many contact and distant healers who believe the source of their healing gift stems from something they believe in, for example, Christianity or Buddhism. There is no requirement that patients should adopt any specific belief, though it is of course preferable that they adopt a positive outlook towards the process of healing. Contact healing is usually conducted through the hands.

At the initial session you will be asked if you have seen your doctor and if not will be recommended to do so. You will be asked why you have come to see the healer, and to give some brief details about your present condition, lifestyle and medical history. There will be no diagnosis. You may be asked to sit in a comfortable chair or lie down on a bed. You may be helped to relax with, for example, soft light such as candlelight and calming music. The healer will sit or stand very near you and take a few minutes to 'attune' to you, passing the hands very near or lightly touching you. The healer will then allow the healing energy to flow through his or her hands to you. You may feel very warm, rather cold, a tingling sensation or a bit dizzy. After treatment you may feel thirsty or drowsy.

One treatment may be enough but sometimes more may be needed. You should talk to your healer about any change in your condition; feedback is very important. The treatment will not interfere with any medication you may be taking.

Limitations and dangers

Although a number of scientific trials have been conducted that clearly suggest some patients/clients benefit from contact healing, there is no guarantee of the effectiveness of healing and no certain explanation of the healing process.

The Confederation of Healing Organizations, the largest group of healing associations in the UK, follows a mandatory and strict code of conduct produced in consultation with the medical establishment. Some of its provisions are set out below. Make sure your healer adheres to them.

THE THERAPIES

- Practitioners shall have respect for the religious, spiritual, political and social views of any individual, irrespective of race, colour, creed or sex.
- Practitioners must never claim to 'cure'. The possible therapeutic benefits may be described: 'recovery' must never be guaranteed.
- Practitioners must not countermand instructions of prescriptions given by a doctor.
- Practitioners must never give a medical diagnosis to a patient/client in any circumstances.
- Practitioners must not use manipulation or vigorous massage unless they possess an appropriate professional qualification.
- Practitioners must not prescribe remedies, herbs, supplements, oils, etc., unless their training and qualifications entitle them to do so.
- Practitioners must act with consideration concerning fees and justification for treatment. (Many healers do not make a charge, or accept donations according to a person's ability to pay.)

Hellerwork

Definition and principles

There are three main components of Hellerwork. The first, deep connective tissue bodywork, is designed to release the tension that currently exists in the connective tissue and to return the body to an aligned position. The second is movement education that promotes body awareness and new movement patterns. The third component is verbal dialogue that focuses on the relationship between emotions, attitudes and the body. The body is restructured with the therapy to restore its fluidity, grace and ease of movement.

Brief outline

Hellerwork was recently developed in the 1970s by an American engineer, Joseph Heller. For a time Heller worked with Ida Rolf (see p. 128). While he agreed with her ideas about body alignment and releasing muscular tension he emphasized the vital importance of the relationship between body and mind and the emotional aspects of this relationship.

Deep tissue manipulation is designed to release accumulated tension in the body's connective tissue that is known as fascia. Fascia is tissue that wraps all the muscles and individual fibres and bundles of individual fibres that become muscle. It comes together at the end of the muscle and becomes the tendon, which attaches the muscle to the bone. Fascia tension can result from physical or emotional trauma and many years of imbalanced movement. A key feature of the therapy is 'guided verbal dialoguing', whereby the patient and practitioner explore emotions that emerge with the release of body tension. It is an integrated system designed to recondition the whole body. The entire musculoskeletal structure of the body is considered and related to the individual's sense of well-being. Changes are seen in relation to the whole body and whole person.

Hellerwork is mainly practised in the USA.

Conditions helped

Hellerwork practitioners claim the following problems may be alleviated using the therapy: back, muscle and neck pain, poor posture, respiratory problems, shoulder pain and sports injuries. Hellerwork is also used to promote health and to prevent postural and stress-related problems. The emphasis, however, is on prevention rather than treatment of illness.

How to find a therapist

There are currently (1999) about 150 practitioners of Hellerwork in the USA but very few elsewhere. For Hellerwork practitioners worldwide, contact the national organization listed on p. 176. If this is not possible, contact a 'general' national organization listed at the beginning of Part IV for further information.

What to expect

At the initial session you will be thoroughly assessed and detailed notes will be made about your lifestyle and medical history. You will be photographed before and after treatment. Each session will concentrate on different areas of the body.

You will become very aware of your body and its pattern of movements and will learn to focus on the use of your body in its daily activities. You will gradually learn about and understand the attitudes and emotional forces that have an affect on your body. Your awareness of these attitudes and emotions will help the process of change. As the tension is released some of the inhibiting patterns of behaviour will also be released.

There are eleven 90-minute sessions. Once you have completed the eleven sessions you will find your body is in a new state of alignment. It will be more balanced and much freer in movement. You will also be much more aware of your bodily needs. Follow-up sessions are available to keep you well balanced in both body and mind.

Limitations and dangers

Hellerwork is not recommended for anyone with high blood pressure, who is overweight, has osteoporosis, rheumatoid arthritis, deep vein thrombosis, shingles, scar tissue, varicose veins or who is pregnant. It is also not recommended for those who bruise easily. There has so far been very little research conducted to prove any benefits.

Herbal medicine – Chinese

Definition and principles

Chinese herbal medicine uses vegetable, mineral and animal products to maintain good health and prevent imbalance of *Qi*. It it used alongside acupuncture (see pp. 28–31). For an account of the basic principles, see Traditional Chinese Medicine (pp. 134–7). The emphasis is on prevention of illness and maintenance of good health rather than curing symptoms. Illness is defined as the individual's struggle to resist disease caused by one or more external factors.

Brief outline

The first known practice of herbalism in China dates back to around 4,500 years ago when a Chinese herbalist listed 365 remedies. By the sixteenth century the practice had become extremely sophisticated, refined and extensive. Li Shi-zhen's *Outline of Materia Medica* listed over 2,000 medicinal plants and 11,000 prescriptions. Today, herbal medicine is available in hospitals throughout China, alongside Western medicine, and is considered to be by far the most important aspect of TCM.

In the UK Chinese herbal medicine has expanded very rapidly throughout the 1990s. This is partly owing to the spectacular results of a trial conducted in 1992 on children suffering severe eczema. These children had not responded to orthodox treatment, but within four weeks of treatment with a formulaic Chinese remedy named Zemaphyte, 60 per cent showed a marked improvement, with no side-effects. When children who did not respond to the formula treatment were given unique treatments according to TCM principles, a further 30 per cent showed a marked improvement.

In the USA there are still many States where the practice of herbal medicine and sale of herbs over the counter are banned. In States where herbal medicine is tolerated, however, such as Montana and New Mexcio, there has very recently been a phenomenal interest and increase in the practice of Chinese herbal medicine. Scientific research is currently being conducted in the USA on the efficacy of many Chinese herbs. Qing Hao (artemisia) has been used as an anti-malarial herb in China for over 2,000 years and recently a scientific study proved its efficacy. Tricosanthin, a Chinese herbal remedy derived from a type of cucumber native to China, and a derivative manufactured in the USA known as GLQ233, have both proved highly effective in treating HIV symptoms, and also very dangerous in certain circumstances.

Conditions helped

There are remedies for every known condition (see TCM, pp. 134–7).

How to find a therapist

It is vital to find a qualified practitioner. As Chinese herbal medicine has only recently been introduced into Western countries, this may be difficult. Contact a national Chinese herbal or TCM organization (see Part IV). If this is not possible, contact a national 'general' organization listed at the beginning of Part IV.

What to expect

The initial consultation will last for at least an hour and you will be very thoroughly examined. The practitioner will ask about your lifestyle, family history, habits, body functions, moods and symptoms. He or she will listen to the tone of your voice and the way you breathe, and will observe the colour of your skin, tongue, hair and the way you move. Your tongue will be looked at and its colour and condition checked to note signs of disease. Your pulse will be taken and the particular rhythms noted. This is claimed to show the condition of internal organs such as the heart, lungs, spleen and kidneys. Areas of discomfort will be gently touched. A diagnosis will be made based on your unique pattern of disharmony and a remedy prescribed. Acupuncture and change of diet may also be advised.

Herbs are rarely prescribed singly. A prescription may include up to 15 herbs. Every herb has a different role to play, with each having one or several functions in a mix of interrelated actions. Practitioners usually adapt a basic formula, adding different herbs to suit the individual's age, character, constitution and particular pattern of disharmony. The mixtures of herbs are often boiled for some time and may be taken as a tea (prepared in daily doses), or pills, powders, pastes, ointments, creams or lotions.

Self treatment

You are advised not to treat yourself with Chinese remedies. Some of the herbs available are dangerous if you overdose. When ginseng first became known in the West it was hailed as a miraculous cure-all, but many people had to go to their doctor because they took too much of this powerful substance. In some instances, people have had to be admitted to hospital after taking certain Chinese remedies, and in a few cases have died from an overdose.

Limitations and dangers

For safety reasons, bear the following points in mind.

- ■ Always consult a qualified practitioner before taking herbal remedies if:
  - you are pregnant or breastfeeding
  - you have high blood pressure, heart disease or glaucoma
  - you are taking prescribed medication.
- ■ Never use herbal remedies if you are suffering from a serious infection, insulin-dependent diabetes, epilepsy or have a serious psychiatric illness such as schizophrenia.
- ■ Never discontinue an allopathically prescribed medicine without telling your doctor.

- Little is known about the interaction of herbal and conventional medicines. Some herbal remedies are known to react badly with particular drugs.
- Not all herbs are safe. There are many Chinese herbs that are very dangerous to take unless they are prescribed and supervised by a qualified practitioner.
- Stop using a herb if you begin to experience any side-effects and contact your Chinese herbal practitioner as soon as possible.
- Never exceed the stated dose.
- Do not take herbal remedies for more than three months consecutively.

There are many Chinese remedies that use parts of animals (and misleadingly come under the label of 'herbal'). Many of the animals, such as tigers, rhinos and bears, are supposed to be protected by the Convention on International Trade in Endangered Species. This, however, does not stop their slaughter and they are rapidly dwindling to the point of extinction. There are many in the West who regard the use of animals for medical purposes to be ethically abhorrent.

Herbal medicine – Western

Definition and principles

Western herbal medicine is the art and science of using plant remedies in the treatment of disease and for ensuring health and well-being. Treatment is holistic with each person being treated as unique. Herbalists are more concerned to look for the cause of illness rather than treat symptoms, as they believe herbal remedies stimulate the body's reaction against illness rather than cure specific problems. They attribute disease to a disruption in the state of harmony in the body, known as homeostasis. This is the 'life force' and the body's self-healing mechanism. They consider the use of herbs, as herbal remedies, encourages the patient's natural recuperative powers by re-establishing the homeostatic balance.

Brief outline

Herbal medicine is probably the oldest system of medicine in the world. Every country has used plants for medicinal purposes and every culture has its own herbal traditions.

Much European knowledge of herbs stemmed from the ancient Greeks and Egyptians, whose priests were also herbal practitioners. During the Middle Ages herbal medicine flourished. Nunneries and monasteries had physic gardens in which medicinal plants were grown, while people were treated for their illnesses in pharmacies and hospitals with remedies obtained from these plants. With the growth of allopathic medicine during the seventeenth century, however, herbal medicine gradually fell out of favour.

In England, herbal medicine was formally established by an Act of Parliament during the reign of Henry VIII. From the early nineteenth century onwards, divisions grew between herbalists. There was a split between the traditional mainly unqualified practitioners and those who insisted on a rigorous academic approach to herbalism. Because of this disunity, herbal medicine did not come under the remit of the National Health Service when it was established in 1948. Nevertheless, it is the only country in Europe where herbalists can practise freely.

In the USA herbal medicine has had a chequered career. It was popular in the late nineteenth century when herbal remedies were used to restore the 'life force', but subsequently went into sharp decline. Much of the revival of interest in the 1970s was owing to D C Jarvis who rediscovered folk remedies in the USA, and to the World Health Organization's report in 1985 which concluded that herbal remedies, the only type of medicine available in most of the developing world, could fulfil an important role in modern health care. In 1994 laws restricting the sale of herbal remedies were relaxed in the USA but even so the practice of medical herbalism is still illegal in many States. In States where it is allowed the practice is suddenly becoming very popular.

International scientific research has confirmed many ancient beliefs about the medicinal properties of plants and incidentally has also widened herbalists' knowledge. Nevertheless, only a small amount of research has been undertaken to confirm or deny the efficacy of plants used for healing. It is estimated there are over three-quarters of a million species of plants that have yet to be examined for possible therapeutic use.

Conditions helped

Herbal remedies have been found to be very instrumental in alleviating problems, in particular the following list of conditions: allergies, arthritis, athlete's foot, baldness, bedwetting, blisters, bruises, burns, candidiasis, common colds, conjunctivitis, croup, cystitis, depression, diarrhoea, digestive problems, diverticulitis, gallstones, hay fever, heavy periods, hives, hyperactivity, insomnia, laryngitis, low blood pressure, menstrual disorders, migraines, mouth ulcers, nausea, neuralgia, obesity, oedema, osteoarthritis, osteoporosis, post-natal depression, psoriasis, respiratory infections, rheumatism, scalds, skin diseases, sore throats, stress-related conditions, thrush, tinnitus, vaginitis, varicose veins, vomiting and warts.

Below are listed some herbs and conditions they are known to alleviate.

- *aloe vera* for healing wounds and improving the blood circulation
- *burdock* for acne
- *camomile* for headaches and vomiting and for healing ulcers and wounds
- *comfrey* for bruises, burns, sprains, strains and wounds
- *cranberry juice* for cystitis
- *elderflower* for fever, influenza and sore throats
- *evening primrose oil* for eczema and pre-menstrual syndrome (PMS)
- *fennel* for flatulence, indigestion, nausea and vomiting
- *fenugreek* for nasal congestion
- *feverfew* for migraine
- *ginko biloba* for blood circulation, loss of memory and tinnitus
- *ginger* for morning and motion sickness, nausea, vomiting and relief from colds and flu
- *liquorice* for gastric ulcers
- *marigold* for cuts, grazes and nappy rash
- *St John's wort* for depression
- *valerian* for anxiety and insomnia.

How to find a therapist

It is essential to find a reputable herbal practitioner who has trained for a minimum of three years full-time or four years part-time. If in doubt consult a national organization (see Part IV). There are many countries where herbal medicine is illegal, and many other countries where anyone can set up as a herbalist without proper training.

What to expect

At the first consultation, which will last for at least an hour, the practitioner will take a full medical history to establish the cause of ill health and also any underlying imbalances. You will probably undergo a physical examination with a blood pressure check and, if deemed useful for diagnostic purposes, have samples of blood and urine taken for analysis, or X-rays. Western herbalists' diagnostic tools and techniques are similar to those of orthodox practitioners, as they are trained in medical diagnosis. You will be asked about your diet, work and family life, your emotional and mental state, whether you have any illnesses and whether you are taking any medication. The herbalist will also evaluate the overall balance of the body's systems to discover underlying disharmonies. Any appropriate prescription will then be dispensed, which may contain a mixture of herbal remedies. Different remedies may be given to treat two people apparently suffering from the same complaint. This is because herbalists treat the whole person, not simply the disease.

You may also be asked to change your lifestyle, particularly diet, to ensure you eat a lot of fruit and fresh vegetables.

You will usually be seen at fortnightly or three-weekly intervals. If you suffer unpleasant side-effects, do not hesitate to contact your herbalist who will vary the prescription to eliminate the offending herb.

Herbal medicine draws on the whole of the plant world for its sources, including shrubs, trees and seaweed. All organs of a plant, such as the rhizome, stem, roots, berries, leaves, bark, flowers or seeds, or even the entire plant, may be used. These contain a mix of active ingredients that produce the plant's medicinal effects. Herbalists claim this mix creates 'synergy', where the therapeutic effect of ingredients is greater when used together rather than separately. They claim plant materials contain a naturally balanced combination of chemicals that reduce the incidence of damaging side-effects. Herbalists argue that using parts of whole plants are more effective than the isolated constituents of plants, such as aspirin from willow bark, used in synthetically made drugs and dispensed by allopathic practitioners. They claim that the active ingredients taken out of context are incompatible with good health.

Plants are harvested and stored, then quickly processed to ensure a high concentration of active ingredients. Remedies may be prescribed in liquid form as tinctures (herbs in alcohol and water), tisanes, fluid extracts or syrups, or they may be given dried to be made into infusions or decoctions. They can also be given as creams, capsules, tablets, ointments, lotions or poultices.

Self treatment

It is unwise to take herbal remedies without consulting a qualified herbal practitioner. There are, however, many over-the-counter remedies in the form of tinctures, creams, tablets or tisanes that you can use to treat common complaints. Always take care to follow instructions on the label and buy products from reputable suppliers.

Limitations and dangers

Always consult a qualified practitioner before taking herbal remedies if:
- you are pregnant or breastfeeding
- you have high blood pressure, heart disease or glaucoma
- you are taking prescribed medication.

For safety reasons, bear the following points in mind.
- Never use herbal remedies if you are suffering from a serious infection, epilepsy or insulin-dependent diabetes, or have a serious psychiatric illness such as schizophrenia.
- Do not collect and use herbs from gardens or the countryside unless you are sure you know what they are and what effect they will have when taken as a remedy.
- Never discontinue an allopathically prescribed medicine without telling your doctor.
- Little is known about the interaction of herbal and conventional medicines. Some herbal remedies are known to react badly with particular drugs. For example kelp (dried seaweed) may interfere with antithyroid drugs.

THE THERAPIES

- Not all herbs are safe. For instance:
  - *bearberry* and *ragwort* can cause liver damage.
  - *broom* and *pennyroyal* can cause miscarriage; broom can also cause jaundice.
  - *comfrey* tablets and capsules can cause liver damage. Comfrey tisanes and creams, however, are not harmful.
  - *feverfew*, if taken raw, can cause mouth ulcers; in tablet form it is not harmful.
  - *mistletoe* can cause gastroenteritis.
- Stop using a herb if you begin to experience any side-effects and go to your herbal practitioner as soon as possible.
- Never exceed the stated dose.
- Do not take herbal remedies for more than three months consecutively.

Homoeopathy

Definition and principles

The word 'homoeopathy' is derived from the Greek 'homoios', meaning like, and 'pathos', meaning suffering.

The major principles of homoeopathic medicine differ from those of orthodox medicine. The therapy is based on the theory that 'like cures like', that is, that a substance that produces the symptoms of a disease may also cure it. This is known as the Law of Similars – 'that which makes sick shall heal'. Another principle is that of the minimum dose. Plant, animal and mineral substances are used to make a remedy and are first soaked in alcohol to extract the active ingredients. This 'mother tincture', as it is called, is progressively diluted many times. There is a vigorous shaking, known as succussion, either by hand or machine, after each dilution. Diluting doses limits the remedy's potential to cause side-effects and it is believed the more a substance is diluted the more potent it becomes. A third principle is the notion of the uniqueness of the remedy, which is regarded as specific to a particular patient at a particular time. A remedy is believed to stimulate the body's immune system and strengthens it against all illness, not one problem only. Homoeopaths do not treat diseases but individuals.

Brief outline

Homoeopathy is based on the beliefs and discoveries of Samuel Hahnemann, a German doctor who trained in orthodox medicine in the late eighteenth century. He gave up his practice in Saxony and experimented with nearly 100 substances that he used on healthy volunteers, incuding himself, his family and friends, and catalogued their effects. Many of the substances were diluted poisons and Hahnemann claimed that small rather than large doses of his remedies would be safer as they would produce fewer side-effects while still remaining effective. He claimed that the more diluted a substance was the more effective it became. Hahnemann also stressed the importance of sensible diet, fresh air, exercise and good hygiene as essential requirements for good health. These were novel and radical ideas at that time. He claimed the first duty of a homoeopath is to effect healing by the safest, quickest, more gentle, most reliable and most permanent means possible.

Over the past 20 years, well over 100 rigorous clinical trials of homoeopathy have been conducted and published and there is now a clear indication that homoeopathic remedies are more than merely placebos. For example, in 1991 the *British Medical Journal* published a review of 107 controlled clinical trials of homoeopathy and found that 77 per cent had positive results. The conditions examined included asthma, pain, respiratory infections and shock. A further study published in the *Lancet* in the UK in 1994 indicated that homoeopathic treatment was more successful than a placebo treatment in relieving asthma and hay fever.

Homoeopathy is very popular in Europe, including the UK (where there are five homoeopathic hospitals under the aegis of the NHS), Australia, New Zealand and India. The therapy is banned in a number of States in the USA but is currently undergoing a revival.

Conditions helped

Homoeopathic remedies can be used to alleviate almost any reversible illness in adults, children and animals. Practitioners have claimed the following conditions have been improved with homoeopathic treatment: acne, agoraphobia, allergies, anaemia, anxiety, arthritis, asthma, baldness (alopecia), Bell's palsy, bladder incontinence, bleeding gums (gingivitis), blisters, boils, bruises, burns, bursitis, catarrh, chilblains, claustrophobia, cold sores, conjunctivitis, constipation, cramp, croup, cystitis, dandruff,

THE THERAPIES

depression, eczema, exhaustion, eye strain, flatulence, gout, grief, halitosis (bad breath), hay fever, headaches, high blood pressure, hives (nettle rash), hyperactivity, hyperventilation, irritable bowel syndrome (IBS), laryngitis, menopausal problems, menstrual problems, migraine, mood swings, morning sickness, myalgic encephalomyelitis (ME), nausea, obesity, panic attacks, peptic ulcers, pre-menstrual syndrome (PMS), psoriasis, shock/trauma, sinusitis, sleep disorders, stress, sweating, rheumatic conditions, teething (babies), tension, tinnitus, tiredness, travel sickness, vomiting, warts and wheezing.

Remedies may be given in hospitals, both before and after operations, to counteract the effects of anxiety, shock and anaesthetic, and also to help with healing. It has been found that many people treated with homoeopathic remedies after operations have made much more rapid post-operative recovery than those who have not received such treatment.

How to find a therapist

It is advisable to find a reputable therapist who is a member of a recognized homoeopathic organization. This may be difficult as there are a number of different branches of homoeopathy, some of which differ considerably in their rationale and treatments. There is also controversy about qualifications required in order to practise the therapy. For instance in the UK there are recognized homoeopaths who have had a full medical training but who have studied homoeopathy for only a short period of time (less than a year). There are other recognized and reputable homoeopaths who have had no medical training but who have had a very thorough grounding in homoeopathy over a period of three or four years. Before having any homoeopathic treatment you are advised to read about the therapy and to consider carefully the type of homoeopathic treatment you think might suit you. Contact one of the national organizations (see Part IV) for further information.

What to expect

The initial session will last for at least an hour, probably longer. The homoeopath will note your likes and dislikes in relation to many factors such as food, climate, people, colours and animals. You will also be asked about your moods and feelings and your hopes, fears and achievements. This is because the homoeopath needs to know as much as possible about you as a whole person; a complete picture has to be built up. You will also be asked about your medical history as well as that of close family members. Once the very thorough investigation has been completed a diagnosis will be made and a remedy prescribed.

The remedy will usually be in the form of a tablet, though it may be a powder, tincture, ointment or even granules. It is believed the remedy stimulates the body's own vital force (homeostasis), the mechanism that generates self healing and helps to achieve a state of equilibrium. If the remedy is in tablet form you will probably be advised to insert it in the mouth and to place it under the tongue to dissolve.

You may find that when you take the remedy you will initially experience what is known as an aggravation reaction, where you will probably feel somewhat worse than you did previously. This, however, usually lasts for only a short time and is never life threatening, though it may be somewhat distressing. Homoeopaths are pleased if there is an aggravation reaction as it is an indication that the remedy is working.

You will probably be recommended not to drink coffee, eat highly spiced food or peppermint or use eucalyptus oil, camphor or methyl while undergoing homoeopathic treatment. The restriction includes the use of many proprietary toothpastes and mouth washes. This is because it is considered that any of these may antidote the effect of the remedy.

At the second and subsequent sessions the therapist will ask you about what has happened since the previous appointment and will check how the remedy is working. A different remedy may be prescribed. The duration of each remedy varies – from hours with acute illnesses to months, years or even a lifetime. As long as the remedy is still working it is important not to take further doses of the same remedy or other remedies.

Self treatment

You can treat yourself using many homoeopathic remedies that are for sale over the counter in pharmacies and health stores. There are two types of remedy: the 'classical' remedy that is named after the single remedy product it contains and the 'indicated' or combined remedy that is usually a combination of three or four remedies that are suitable for treating a particular problem (like orthodox medicine). Note, however, that a remedy bought over the counter is not made to suit you specifically at a particular time. As such it is unlikely to be of much benefit.

Limitations and dangers

Although there have been many scientific trials which have demonstrated that homoeopathy has been effective in alleviating a wide range of conditions, the therapy is nevertheless regarded with suspicion by most orthodox practitioners. Claims made by homoeopathic practitioners, particularly with regard to curing ailments, are not usually accepted by the medical profession.

It is important to take note of the following:

- Homoeopathic remedies can cause an initial aggravation, which is usually a good sign. If this happens, stop taking the remedy and consult your homoeopath.
- Although a lot of problems may be alleviated using one remedy and with one treatment only, many conditions require treatments with different remedies over a long period of time.
- Check any unexplained symptoms with a doctor if you are consulting a non-medically trained homoeopath after you have reported them to your homoeopath.
- Certain essential oils are not compatible with homoeopathic treatment. If you are using essential oils, tell your homoeopath about them.
- If you are allergic to milk-based products, ask for lactose-free homoeopathic remedies.

Hydrotherapy

Definition and principles

Hydrotherapy is using water, either externally or internally, to cleanse and revitalize the body and maintain or restore health.

Brief outline

Water has many healing properties. Hot water dilates the blood vessels that reduce blood pressure while increasing blood flow to the muscles, thereby easing stiffness. Cold water stimulates and invigorates both mind and body. Hot and cold water are often used in conjuction.

Conditions helped

Hydrotherapy is particularly effective for alleviating discomforts associated with spinal stress and for those with varicose veins. It also helps with burn injuries, coughs, croup, cystitis, headaches, menstrual problems, rheumatoid arthritis and sinusitis.

How to find a therapist

Hydrotherapists are hard to find. Contact one of the national hydrotherapy, naturopathic or osteopathic organizations listed in Part IV.

What to expect

There are hot, cold, whirlpool, sweating, aerated and Sitz baths. High powered jets with strong streams or sprays of water stimulate the circulation and ease muscular pain. Jacuzzis are used in hospitals to relieve pressure sores and for bedridden patients. Colonic irrigation, consisting of water at body temperature being injected into the rectum, clears the colon of poisons, gas, accumulated faecal matter and mucous deposits. Thalassotherapy uses sea water or seaweed that induces sweating, thus cleansing and toning the skin and lymphatic system. Coughs, croup and sinus problems are helped by inhaling steam vapours through the nose from water to which various essential oils have been added.

Self treatment

You can use hot compresses to ease back or abdominal pain and muscle tension. An ice pack relieves pain and swelling in emergencies. Place a towel or a drop of oil on the skin to avoid a freezer burn, then apply ice or a packet of frozen peas wrapped in a cloth to the affected area. Leave for ten minutes.

Limitations and dangers

Hydrotherapy is not recommended for people with high blood pressure, angina or heart disease. Avoid if you are pregnant. Do not have steam treatments if you have recently had a major operation or are epileptic, asthmatic or have a history of thrombosis. Avoid any seaweed treatment if you are allergic to iodine.

Hypnotherapy

Definition and principles

Hypnotherapy, often referred to as the art of suggestion, is a method of healing using hypnosis to tap into the unconscious to achieve behavioural change. Hypnosis is a state of altered consciousness during which the unconscious mind, which controls autonomic bodily responses, becomes receptive to suggestion. To observers, people under hypnosis appear to be sleeping, but they are awake and aware of what is going on. The awareness experienced, however, is different from that experienced in an ordinary conscious state. For people under hypnosis, the reality of the external world is relegated to the back of their minds while they experience increased receptivity and responsiveness to suggestions received from therapists.

Brief outline

The therapy has existed for many thousands of years. The Sumerians and Egyptians practised hypnosis for healing, as well as holy men in ancient India and Persia. The father of modern hypnotherapy was Dr James Braid (1795–1860), who used hypnotism when operating on patients in hospitals in Manchester, England, in the nineteenth century. He suggested that the physical relaxation and altered conscious awareness state entered into by patients should be called hypnotism, from the Greek *hypnos* meaning sleep, as they seemed to be in a sleep-like state.

Although Braid achieved excellent results with his treatments and although there were many other eminent physicians, including Freud, who used hypnosis successfully, it was not until comparatively recently that the therapy became acceptable to use. In the UK in 1893 a British Medical Association (BMA) committee mentioned hypnotism favourably, stating that 'as a therapeutic agent hypnotism is frequently effective in relieving pain, procuring sleep and alleviating many functional ailments'. It was only in 1955, however, that a second BMA report on hypnotism approved its use for the treatment of psychoneuroses and for the relief of pain. It also recommended that all doctors and medical students should receive adequate training in its application.

Conditions helped

Hypnotherapy has been found to be very useful in treating a variety of problems. It has proved effective in eliminating addictive behaviour such as smoking, alcoholism or gambling, and in helping to cure undesirable habits such as nail-biting or teeth-grinding. It has also proved effective in treating certain states of depression and anxiety as well as phobias (fear of open spaces, lifts, tunnels, etc.). Another success has been in helping people to control their weight and in treating eating disorders such as anorexia and bulimia. It has been used as a psychotherapeutic tool to control pain; in dentistry the technique is used for analgesia if patients are allergic to anaesthetics. The therapy has been successful in treating physical conditions where there is a psychological element, for example, psychosomatic illnesses such as hysterical paralysis or kleptomania, or conditions caused by stress such as bedwetting, eczema, psoriasis or irritable bowel syndrome (IBS). In addition, hypnotherapy has proved useful for those who want to enhance their personal development, such as increasing performance in a particular sport, or in their work or memory.

How to find a therapist

It is very important indeed to find a reputable hypnotherapist. If in any doubt about whom to contact, you should liaise with one of the national organizations listed in Part IV rather than rely on the advice of friends or relatives who may have only heard about someone through friends of their own, rather than having had treatment themselves. Third-hand advice is very often unreliable. In most countries there are no restrictions on setting up as a hypnotherapist and there is no statutory control. In the UK, for instance, anyone can place an advertisement offering hypnotherapy. Certificates and diplomas can be obtained without any legal check; and anyone can set up a training school.

What to expect

At the first session the practitioner will take detailed notes about your medical history and lifestyle. Particular attention will be paid to your present problems and to past treatment given by other medical or alternative practitioners. You should be given a full explanation of what hypnotherapy entails and what will happen to you when you undergo treatment. A brief account of what happens is set out below.

Your attention will be directed inwards and you will learn to concentrate on suggestions given by your therapist. These suggestions will often be in the form of images. You will feel relaxed and reluctant to move, will breathe more slowly, will flutter your eyelids and, under hypnosis, will almost certainly lose a sense of time. (Once out of the hypnotic state you are most likely to find you have considerably underestimated the time spent in a trance.)

Extensive research has shown that while about 10 per cent of people worldwide can be hypnotized very easily, 10 per cent are very difficult to hypnotize. The majority, 80 per cent, can be hypnotized without too much difficulty. It is important to remember, however, that no one can be hypnotized against his or her will. Your mind will not be interfered with and neither will your personality change under hypnosis. You will not be forced to do or say things that are against your will or that you don't want to speak about. The therapist may implant suggestions that may be triggered after you come out of the hypnotic state but if you are unwilling to follow these up you are not forced to do so. Contrary to what is commonly believed, the patient never loses control and some part of the mind is always aware of what is being said and done, so you will almost certainly remember what happens after you come out of the hypnotic trance.

It is very important for both the patient and practitioner to build up a rapport with, and to trust, each other at the initial session, otherwise treatment will not be successful and might well be damaging to the patient.

It is unlikely that hypnosis will be used at the first session. You will, however, be assessed for the type of therapy required. There are three main types of hypnotherapy: suggestion therapy, desensitization therapy and analytical hypnotherapy.

With suggestion therapy the practitioner gives suggestions, in words and images, to the patient to help change bad habits, negative image and low performance levels. Problems helped include stress, eating disorders, bedwetting, insomnia, negative self-image and sexual problems.

Desensitization therapy helps patients cope with fears and phobias. Situations that arouse fear or phobia are very gradually introduced to the patient under hypnosis until they no longer create an intense reaction. The practitioner will ensure the patient remains calm throughout treatment and will slowly build up the patient's confidence by very gradually introducing more and more advanced steps. Desensitization therapy helps with fear and phobias such as fear of flying, crowds, spiders, snakes, illness, being alone, enclosed spaces, being outside and heights.

Analytical therapy has as its objective to discover the underlying reason for a problem. The cause of the problem will be worked through to make the symptom(s) redundant. Re-experiencing past traumas under hypnosis, known as abreaction, helps to release pent-up emotions and helps the patient to let go of the trauma. Analytical therapy is used to help eliminate addictive behaviours, anxiety, asthma, depression, eating disorders, eczema, obsessions or compulsions and panic attacks or phobias.

Self treatment

You can treat yourself for some conditions. You become your own therapist and learn to use the power of your subconscious mind to influence the way you behave. Self-hypnosis helps with recovery after an illness; it can build up self-confidence; can enhance creativity; can help with weight control, tension headaches and insomnia.

It is essential that you go to a reputable therapist who will teach you the correct techniques for self-hypnosis. This is very important as it is difficult to learn to hypnotize oneself correctly without professional help. If you don't learn the techniques properly, you might well be creating more problems than you are solving. You will learn from a therapist to set a goal and to get together a number of positive suggestions to help you reach this goal. You must be positive throughout and learn repetitive techniques. You will learn from your therapist how to induce self-hypnosis and how to give yourself the required suggestions. If you learn properly, and this does take time, self-hypnosis can prove remarkably effective, partly because you only have yourself to worry about; there is no one else involved. Once you have decided you really want to employ this technique and then learn how to do so properly, there should be no major problem.

Limitations and dangers

As emphasized above, it is very important indeed to find a reputable hypnotherapist. In addition, it is suggested that hypnotherapy should not be used for people who suffer from epilepsy or who are psychotic, for example, suffering from schizophrenia. It has also been suggested that hypnotherapy should not be used for sufferers of symptomatic or manic depression as the hypnotherapeutic techniques used are very similar to the symptoms shown in these types of depression.

Iridology

Definition and principles

Iridology uses the eyes, particularly the irises, to assess states of health and well-being. The condition, pigmentation, structure and marking of the irises, which are unique to each individual, are studied in depth. With regular check-ups over a period of time, changes are carefully noted. Iridology is a diagnostic technique and form of monitoring health, not a therapy, and claims to detect changes in the eyes before they manifest in the physical body.

Brief outline

Throughout Europe from the seventeenth century onwards, diagnosing the state of an individual's health using an examination of the eyes became an established medical practice. It is, however, a Hungarian doctor, Ignatz von Peczely, who is regarded as the originator of iridology. He believed the eye's iris was an indicator of potential organic disease. Specific diseased organs, he claimed, could be highlighted by being able to diagnose conditions residing within the iris. He published numerous papers relating to his theories in the late nineteenth century, but following his death in 1911 his work was largely ignored for nearly half a century. During the 1950s, however, an American physician, Dr Bernard Jensen, developed von Peczely's work and produced a more detailed map of each iris. Today these maps have been further refined and iridologists claim they can detect not only past but also potential physical and psychological problems.

It is thought there are three main constitutional types of individuals, determined by eye colour:

- *lymphatic*, with mainly blue or blue grey eyes, with a tendency towards conditions such as arthritis, rheumatism, catarrh and upper respiratory problems
- *haematogenous*, with dark brown eyes, with a tendency towards anaemia, a slow metabolic rate, glandular disturbances and blood disorders
- *biliary*, with a mixture of blue, brown and hazel eyes, with a tendency towards weak digestion and diseases of the gall-bladder and liver.

Iridologists claim that the organs and tissues throughout the body are reflected through the fibres and thousands of fine nerve filaments of the irises, which form patterns showing tissue change in the iris before it becomes diseased. When in good health the colours of the iris are bright, clear and vibrant. Poor health, however, is reflected by iris discoloration. By detecting and analysing tissue changes, an iridologist can recommend a suitable therapy or change in lifestyle, particularly diet, to help prevent disease.

Iridologists produce very detailed maps of each iris, which is divided into radial segments corresponding to different parts or functions of the body. Many parts or functions are reflected in both irises. It is thought the left eye registers changes in the left side of the body while the right eye shows changes in the right side.

Conditions helped

Iridologists claim to be able to diagnose most conditions. They do not pinpoint or treat specific diseases. What they claim to do is identify physical weaknesses and underlying health problems, such as hardening of the arteries. These may lead, or may have already led, to disease. To treat a problem, most iridologists recommend other complementary or alternative therapies, particularly naturopathy, herbal medicine or some form of massage. Those who do not like invasive diagnostic techniques of conventional medicine, such as blood tests, X-rays and biopsies may prefer the non-invasive eye examinations. Note, however, that there is as yet no scientific evidence for validity of diagnosis. Those who want to keep a check on their health and well-being and who want advance warning of possible disease might well benefit from this practice.

How to find a therapist

It is essential to find a qualified practitioner. Before deciding to have a consultation, enquire about the practitioner's training and whether or not he or she has been trained in anatomy or physiology. Make sure that if you are diagnosed as having a problem the iridologist will be able to refer you to a qualified practitioner in a suitable alternative therapy. If in any doubt, consult your doctor. Contact one of the national organizations listed in Part IV.

THE THERAPIES

What to expect

You have to remove glasses or contact lenses before diagnosis. Practitioners may use a torch, magnifying glass, ophthalmoscope or an iroscope. The latter is a special video camera with a close-up lens and side lighting used to photograph the irises for a permanent record. It projects the enlarged image of the eyes on to a large screen for analysis. A detailed record of the marking on the irises will be made. The condition of the iris will be closely examined as well as the fibres radiating from the pupil. Your iridologist will explain the significance of the various markings. Subsequently you will be recommended a suitable alternative therapist or allopathic practitioner who will treat the problem diagnosed. You will require one or two sessions for a detailed diagnosis and then follow-up sessions at regular intervals to check on improvements in your state of health and general well-being.

Limitations and dangers

Although iridology is not harmful, most orthodox practitioners consider it to be a misleading diagnostic tool. Clinical trials have so far indicated that iridology has for the most part failed to diagnose disease, and ophthalmologists do not recognize iridology as having any place in medicine. Epileptics should not undergo iridology as the bright lights used for diagnosis may trigger a fit. It is not suitable for any serious infection or any serious condition that might be caused by underlying disease.

Kinesiology

Definition and principles

Kinesiology is based on the notion that there are meridians (energy channels) (see TCM p. 135) for body organs and muscles. Weaknesses in specific muscles indicate potential illnesses or help to diagnose existing imbalances. It is thought that toxins build up and collect in tissues around acupoints. The toxins create discomfort and cause problems that affect muscles surrounding these pressure points.

Brief outline

A recent therapy, kinesiology was created by an American chiropractor, Dr George Goodhart, in the 1960s.

Conditions helped

Kinesiology is used to detect muscle weaknesses, back and neck pains, incorrect joint function and spinal lesions. It has been found to help reduce sciatica, headaches, indigestion and depression. Kinesiology has also been found useful for detecting allergies, particularly food allergies. The therapy is widely used in chiropractic and osteopathic practices in the USA, Australasia and Europe.

How to find a therapist

Information about therapists can be obtained from all major kinesiology organizations (see Part IV). A reputable kinesiologist should have trained for at least two years and undertaken at least 200 hours of kinesiology.

What to expect

At the first session a practitioner takes a detailed history of your lifestyle and illnesses. You may be asked to change your diet and to exercise more frequently. Your gait and posture will be examined before the practitioner tests the strength and mobility of certain muscles. Weak muscles will indicate a particular problem to the therapist who will then gently massage appropriate acupoints on the body or scalp. This treatment will revitalize the flow of energy, strengthen weakened muscles and disperse the build-up of poisons. You should feel better quickly after treatment, which may take up to one-and-a-half hours.

Limitations and dangers

Although there are many who claim to have benefited from kinesiology, orthodox medical practitioners remain sceptical.

Light therapy

Definition and principles

Light therapy is healing through exposure to sunlight or the use of either ultraviolet (UV) light or very bright artificial light.

Conditions helped

Ultraviolet light has helped cure tuberculosis and its antiviral, antibacterial and antifungal properties have benefited those with skin problems such as eczema and psoriasis. Bright artificial light has helped people suffering from depression, high blood pressure, insomnia, seasonal affective disorder (SAD) and those who have disturbed sleep patterns because of jet lag or working night shifts. Light therapy may also help with women's infertility as it stimulates ovulation.

How to find a therapist

Contact one of the national organizations listed in Part IV for a qualified therapist.

What to expect

The usual treatment consists of lying on a bed with your eyes open for up to an hour at a time, under a lamp emitting full-spectrum or bright white light of at least 2,500 lux. This is at least twice the light experienced in offices (between 500 and 1,000 lux), but still only half the average amount of light in daylight (5,000 lux). UV treatment is somewhat different and lasts for less time.

If you suffer from SAD you should take daily exercise outside during daylight hours and also buy a light box to use at home each day during the winter months. (Over 70 per cent of SAD sufferers who have used light boxes regularly have found relief from their symptoms.) Light boxes emit either full-spectrum light (equivalent to natural sunlight) or a very bright light that does not include UV rays.

Limitations and dangers

It is essential to avoid overexposure to UV light as this can cause skin cancer. If you are having light therapy treatment do not take vitamin D supplements as high doses are toxic. Do not undergo light therapy if you have any eye disorder or allergies that might be exacerbated by treatment. Always check with a properly qualified light therapy practitioner before embarking on any form of light therapy.

Massage

Definition and principles

Massage, using stroking and kneading techniques, relaxes and revives the body and mind physically, mentally and emotionally.

Brief outline

Massage as a healing technique has been known for at least 3,000 years and ancient physicians used the therapy effectively in treating fatigue, illness and injury.

In the West today there are around 100 different types of massage. It is often used in conjunction with other therapies, particularly with aromatherapy (see pp. 36–41), osteopathy (see pp. 112–16) and chiropractic (see pp. 59–63), in re-establishing and maintaining the postural integrity of the body.

Most present-day techniques derive from what is known as Swedish or Classical massage. During the nineteenth century in Sweden, Henrik Ling demonstrated the physical and psychological benefits of particular techniques. He rationalized the many different strokes then used. Swedish massage was praised and the benefits of massage acknowledged by orthodox practitioners; during the First World War it was used to treat victims of shell-shock. Later, however, the popularity of massage waned as electrical instruments rather than manual methods were used to treat the human body. Also, its reputation suffered because of the popular association with dubious sexual activities and massage parlours. However, since George Downing published his *Massage Book* in the early 1970s and reiterated the importance of massage and human touch as a healing technique, massage has gradually regained its former status as a mechanism for healing.

Various forms of touch are applied to the muscles and ligaments of the body and are designed both to relax, and strengthen and stimulate. Practitioners say that massage benefits both the masseur and the person being massaged as both touching and being touched create positive psychological advantages. There are many proven benefits. Massage helps to relieve pain, free and mobilize stiff joints and aids recovery from minor soft tissue problems. It enables the digestive system to function efficiently. It is known to ease tensions and knotted tissue, increase the circulation of the blood and stimulate the lymphatic system which helps to eliminate waste material. There may be a reduction in anxiety as a result of lower cortisone levels. Massage reduces swollen tissues by encouraging lymphatic drainage and helps to break down adhesions and restore strength and mobility after injury. It relieves pain, and not only reduces the subjective effects of pain and lessens spasm but releases endorphins, the body's natural sedatives. In 1995 research at the Royal Marsden Hospital in London proved conclusively that massage improved life for cancer patients by substantially reducing stress and anxiety.

Conditions helped

Massage brings about a feeling of well-being and stability. It has been used to alleviate and sometimes eliminate the following conditions: aching joints, anorexia nervosa, anxiety, back pain, Bell's palsy, bulimia nervosa, bursitis, catarrh, chilblains, circulation problems, constipation, cramp, dandruff, depression, feeling run down, fibrositis, fluid retention, frozen shoulder, headaches, hip disorders, hyperactivity, indigestion, insomnia, irritable bowel syndrome (IBS), jet lag, joint problems, lumbago, myalgic encephalomyelitis (ME), menopausal problems, migraine, mood swings, muscle stiffness, neck pain, nervous disorders, palpitations, panic attacks, post-natal depression, pre-menstrual syndrome (PMS), repetitive strain injury (RSI), rheumatism, shock, sinusitis, soft tissue injuries, sports injuries, stress and teeth grinding.

How to find a therapist

It is very important to choose a qualified practitioner who has thoroughly learnt and mastered the techniques. A masseur who doesn't really know what to do can quite easily cause harm to muscles and ligaments. Your doctor may be able to provide you with the name of a qualified practitioner, otherwise consult a national organization (see Part IV).

What to expect

You lie down on a firm surface in a warm room, naked except for underwear, and partially covered by a towel. The masseur will show you how to lie.

The Swedish massage outlined above incorporates four basic techniques.

- *Effleurage* comprises slow, rhythmic gliding strokes, with the masseur using the palms, fingertips and ball of the thumb. An expanse of skin, such as the forearm or thigh, may be stroked with fingers relaxed, using the whole surface of the palm of the hand. Effleurage is the background to all other strokes and is used at the beginning and end of a session. It is a gentle massage and does not put any pressure on the body.
- *Percussion* consists of sharp, fast and stimulating movements that are usually delivered with the side of the hand to strengthen and tone muscles. *Tapotement* is the lightest percussion massage, usually applied to sensitive areas around the face and head. *Hacking*, performed lightly with the fingers, makes muscles 'wake up' without your sense of being relaxed becoming disturbed. *Cupping*, used on the lower back and over the rib cage, prepares the large muscles for action.
- *Friction* or *frottage* is deep massage using the thumbs, fingers or heel of the hand in a series of small, circular movements. It helps to ease muscle tension and improve the blood and lymph circulation. It is used to treat damaged or strained ligaments and tendons and helps free stiff and locked joints.
- *Petrissage* is deep, sometimes painful, massage where the flesh is kneaded and squeezed between finger and thumb. This helps to relax contracted muscles and improve circulation. The kneading may also be done with the heel of the hand or foot, knuckles or elbow. The experience of being kneaded can be very emotional as deep tensions are released.

Self treatment

It is easy to massage parts of your own body, but this is not nearly so relaxing – or stimulating – as being massaged by someone else. A partner may give you a light massage on the back of the neck or shoulders, but for deep massage an experienced practitioner is recommended. Always ensure that both you and your masseur talk about what you want before beginning the massage.

Limitations and dangers

Massage is not suitable for any conditions that may be caused by serious underlying disease. It is also not suitable for women in early pregnancy (that is, under three months); those suffering from infectious diseases; those with deep vein thrombosis, shingles, varicose veins, phlebitis or heart disease. It is also unsuitable for those who are suffering from the inflammatory stage of arthritis.

Medical astrology

Definition and principles

The planets and signs of the zodiac are seen in terms of physiology and anatomy, and may indicate diseases and remedies. Rather than providing a medical diagnosis or cure, the root cause of disease is identified. It is assumed that each individual is unique, and that the body, emotions, mind and spirit are completely interdependent; the homeostatic process inherent in each individual plays a very important role in prevention and treatment of illness; individuals should know about and be active in their treatment.

Brief outline

Medical astrologers claim astrology can provide insights relating to the diagnosis, prognosis and most effective treatment for individuals and their illnesses. Some use their patient's natal chart, based on the individual's date and place of birth, while others use the Decumbiture method. With the latter the practitioner sets up a chart related specifically for the time of the illness enquired about.

Conditions helped

Medical astrology practitioners may be consulted about all known diseases. They will not treat *per se* but will provide insight into the genesis of the illness and indicate avenues of cure.

How to find a therapist

It is vital to choose a medical astrologer who has a thorough grounding in astrology. He or she should have a balanced personality, interpersonal skills and be experienced in psychological and spiritual processes.

What to expect

The problem areas need to be located and defined using various astrological techniques. You will be helped to become aware of and to understand your physical and mental states and how these affect your being. You will be encouraged to use a medium that you feel predisposed towards, such as talking, writing, drawing or dancing to help you to express your feelings and thoughts as a prelude to the healing process.

Medical astrologers use various remedies to help with healing, such as herbs, homoeopathic and flower remedies, acupuncture, colour and sound.

Limitations and dangers

Medical astrology is far removed from science and the objective world of proof and facts. There are very few orthodox practitioners who accept the way it works.

Meditation

Definition and principles

Meditation is a process of relaxation and concentration leading to contemplation. It is used to focus the mind, relax and balance bodily processes. Most people who use the various techniques employed aim to reach a tranquil, relaxed state, inner harmony and increased awareness of both themselves and their environment.

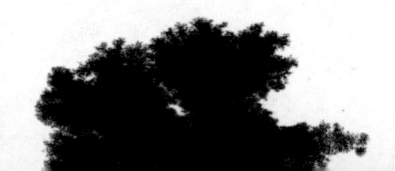

Brief outline

Meditation has been practised for thousands of years, particularly in Asia and India where the techniques have been used as methods for personal growth and self-realization with the aim of reaching spiritual enlightenment. In Western countries today, many orthodox as well as alternative practitioners accept the importance of meditation for achieving a balance between mind, feelings and body. It has been shown to help realign the body's homeostatic mechanism with its calming effect on brainwave patterns, the autonomic nervous system and higher centres in the cerebral cortex. During meditation, breathing, brain activity, heart and pulse rate slow down.

There are many techniques used by schools of meditation to help achieve the ideal state of 'passive awareness'. Some of these are listed below.

- *Breathing exercises* are used in Buddhist meditation, known as *Vipassana*, and in hatha yoga as *pranayama*. This seeks to change negative states of mind such as hatred, sloth and anger into positive thoughts, radiating, for instance, joy, peace and contentment. The aim is to enter a state of 'diffuse openness', aware of, but detached from, everything you are experiencing. Vipanssana uses breathing exercises to develop an awareness of breathing and positive feelings.

- *Concentration* may be helped by concentrating on a specific topic, for example, contemplation of a *mandala*, a spiritual painting in geometric form. Other types of sensory stimulation are also used, such as a picture of a guru or a candle flame. Sometimes concentration is helped by stimulating the sense of smell using relaxing aromatic oils or burning special incense.

- *Chanting*, for example, *mantras*, which are sacred words or phrases. Mantras occupy the mind and the vibration of sound helps to concentrate energy. Transcendental meditation, taught in the 1960s by Maharishi Mahesh Yogi, requires its adherents to sit comfortably with eyes closed repeating a mantram for about 20 minutes a day.

- *Movement exercises* such as t'ai chi (see p. 132), qigong (see p. 120), or hatha yoga (see p. 141).

Research undertaken in the USA in 1992 has shown that Vipassana (see above) can reduce anxiety, panic attacks and agoraphobia. Other studies have shown conclusively that meditation can reverse the effects of stress.

Conditions helped

Meditation has been found to help alleviate and sometimes eliminate the following problems: addictions, agoraphobia, anxiety, asthma, chest complaints, circulation problems, conditions associated with heart disease, depression, fatigue, female and male frigidity, heartburn, high blood pressure, hypertension, indigestion, insomnia, irritable bowel syndrome (IBS), myalgic encephalomyelitis (ME), menopause, migraine, muscular tension, nausea, panic attacks, peptic ulcers, phobias, post-natal depression, pre-menstrual syndrome (PMS), shock, stress-related problems and tension.

People who meditate claim they are better able to cope with everyday problems and stresses and suffer fewer illnesses. They learn how to become more self-confident and achieve a strong sense of self. It is claimed they become much more sensitive to the environment in which they live, and also recover much more quickly from a stressful situation once it has passed. Also, less sleep is required by those who meditate regularly.

How to learn to meditate

There are a few people who are able to learn how to meditate on their own without the need of a teacher but most of us need help to begin with. You are strongly advised to go to an accredited school of meditation to learn some basic techniques.

Meditation requires time, concentration and persistence. The following are some basic suggestions to help you meditate. It has to be reiterated, however, that you should go to an accredited teacher to receive proper guidance before trying to learn anything by yourself. A teacher will tell you about the techniques and how to practise them.

Do not eat or drink for half an hour before beginning to meditate. Choose a room where you will not be interrupted. Sit comfortably, with your back straight and shoulders relaxed, preferably with your eyes open so that you are not tempted to fall asleep. Rest your hands on your lap or on your thighs so your shoulders are loose. To help stop troubling or stimulating thoughts, breathe deeply and concentrate on breathing in through the nose, so that your breath fills your lungs completely. Hold your breath for a few seconds while the lungs are full, then slowly exhale. Repeat this ten times.

You should now be alert and in control of your body and mind, ideally in a state of 'passive awareness'. While you are meditating, breathe slowly and rhythmically. Be aware of the tense parts of your body and try to imagine loosening all your muscles. Stay as still as you possibly can, even if you get an itch or feel a bit of cramp; these irritations may well fade away. Try not to let your mind wander and allow your attention to be directed inwards, beyond mental activity, to an awareness of your inner self. You should be focused entirely in the present, in a state of 'balanced passivity', and not be troubled or excited by past memories or future anxieties. If it helps, concentrate on your heartbeat, or something you can see around you, or visualize an object such as a rose.

When you want to finish, take time to become fully aware of your surroundings. Stretch and stand up slowly. At first, don't try to meditate for more than ten minutes at a time, and never more than twice a day. You should, however, meditate at least once a day. You can gradually increase the meditation time to half an hour.

Limitations and dangers

Meditation is not recommended for people who have a history of mental illness, such as schizophrenia. It will not help with serious infections or any condition that might be caused by serious underlying disease. Very occasionally, people who meditate become disorientated and confused. If this happens you are advised to discontinue the practice at once.

Metamorphic technique

Definition and principles

The metamorphic technique consists of light massage to reflexes in the head, hands and feet. The aim is to release physical and emotional blocks established during the pre-natal period and to foster creative and positive changes in our lives.

Brief outline

The therapy was developed by a British naturopath, Robert St John, during the 1960s while he was working in a school for children with learning difficulties. St John believed the most important time in our lives is the pre-natal period and claimed that who we are emotionally, mentally and physically is predetermined or patterned while we are still in the womb, and that the diet, feelings and thoughts of the mother pattern the foetus. It is a fundamental tenet of the technique that the state of a pregnant woman's mind can affect the future health of the unborn child. He posited that health is wholeness, a free-flowing of life-energy without impediment. If, however, the life-energy is blocked, perhaps through some trauma in the womb, it may result in physical, emotional, mental or spiritual illness.

The metamorphic technique focuses on the relationship between the feet and the growth of the baby in the womb. Working on spinal reflex points of the feet, hands and head helps the individual to loosen and escape from the restrictive patterns set up during the gestation period. Practitioners claim that by lightly touching areas along an imaginary line running from the ankle along the arch to the big toe as well as parts of the hands and head, they can free a person's 'life force', which in turn can alter negative patterns laid down in the past that is, pre-birth.

Practitioners do not make any comments or offer counselling, because they claim the actual healing is done by the patient.

Conditions helped

No claims are made to cure any ailment but the technique does aim to facilitate a positive approach to life by encouraging 'transformations' that loosen old ways of thinking and behaving, and allow new ones to take their place. Practitioners claim the therapy benefits those with autism and Down's syndrome, as well as children with learning difficulties. The technique may act as a catalyst in allowing the innate life force to bring about healing. The technique is reckoned to help treat addictions because it encourages a person's 'vital energy' to fight drugs and at the same time restores lost self-esteem.

It is claimed the patient gains inner strength and self-esteem because it is the patient who is effecting the healing and making a 'transformation'.

How to find a therapist

There are very few practitioners of the metamorphic technique. Contact a national organization for a reputable practitioner. If there are no national organizations, contact one of the 'general' organizations listed at the beginning of Part IV.

What to expect

Unlike most alternative therapies, you will not be asked about your lifestyle or health or be given dietary advice. You will sit comfortably, having removed shoes and socks. Both feet are massaged gently by the practitioner who will use light, circular movements. Later, the hands and head will also be massaged.

Often you will not feel anything at all but sometimes after a session you may feel very relaxed or feel 'electrical' type sensations flowing through the body.

Each session usually lasts for about an hour.

Limitations and dangers

No harm can be caused, provided the technique is used correctly. Orthodox practitioners are in the main sceptical about any benefits. It is impossible to test for the technique's effectiveness.

Music therapy

Definition and principles

Music evokes mood, sensation and emotion and provides a bridge between the conscious and unconscious mind.

Brief outline

Pythagoras used music to heal 'soul sickness'. Modern music therapy developed in the USA at the end of the Second World War out of music played to help war veterans suffering psychological distress.

Conditions helped

Those recovering from illness or an operation recover more quickly and feel less anxiety and discomfort if they listen to quiet music. Music with certain rhythms may reduce stress by lowering heart-rate, blood pressure and respiration. Used for rehabilitation purposes and for those who are terminally ill, it helps those who cannot communicate verbally. Music has helped mentally disturbed people, psychotics and hyperactive children or children with learning difficulties, such as autism and Down's syndrome. It has also benefited those suffering from acute depression, stress or anxiety.

How to find a therapist

It is very important to choose a fully qualified therapist, that is, a trained musician with a degree and postgraduate qualification in music therapy. Contact a national organization (see Part IV).

What to expect

You do not need to be musical and the therapy is said to work however crude the music. In fact it is said to work better if you make the music yourself. You can either listen to music alone or as part of a group, improvise sounds or play instruments to build up confidence and self-esteem with a view to facing inner conflicts. You are given the choice of what to do and encouraged to choose your own methods of making music. The therapist's role is to encourage, observe what happens and assess the psychotherapeutic process.

Self treatment

You can treat yourself by listening to music every day – you probably do so already! But a qualified therapist is necessary to help to express and evaluate emotions, moods and sensations that perhaps have been blocked for many years.

Limitations and dangers

Be aware of deep emotions that may be released by music therapy and make sure you have a fully qualified therapist to guide you.

Naturopathy

Definition and principles

Naturopathy, also known as natural medicine or nature cure, is based on the idea of the body's ability to cure itself. It emphasizes a way of life in harmony with nature and aims to encourage health by supporting and stimulating nature's healing power to maintain or regain health and balance. Naturopaths claim the body will always strive towards equilibrium, that is, health.

Naturopaths believe disease is brought about by an imbalance in the body and that illness affects the whole person – the mind, emotions, body and spirit. A naturopath's aim is to bring the body back to the point where it can heal itself. It supports the vital principle known as *Qi*, *prana*, or homeostasis.

The discipline is based on four principles:

- the individual is unique
- there is a need to treat the whole person, not simply the area of the body affected by disease
- it is more important to establish the cause of the condition than to treat the symptoms
- individuals have the power to heal themselves.

Naturopaths never claim to cure, only treat. They believe that only nature can cure, and that fresh air, water, exercise and a balanced diet of fresh foods are the foundation of good health.

There are four distinct aspects of the healing process:

- the self-healing mechanisms of the body known as the 'vital force' or homeostasis
- the capacity of the organism to activate its self-healing mechanisms in response to treatment, known as heterostasis
- disease is a manifestation of the body's inherent power applying itself to remove obstructions to the normal functioning of organs and tissues
- there is a tendency for the organism recovering from chronic disease to pass through more acute phases, a process known as the Law of Cure. A fever or rash is seen as a way of re-establishing health. Because a fever increases the metabolic rate and accelerates the circulation of the blood, toxins can be eliminated more quickly.

Brief outline

The philosophical basis of naturopathy dates back to Hippocrates (c. 460–375 BC) who emphasized nature's healing powers and the use of naturally occurring medicines in foods. Good health, he claimed, is based on eating and exercising in moderation. It is only nature that heals, provided it is given the opportunity to do so. Disease is a way of purifying the body. Fasting allows the body to deal with disease and eliminates digestion.

Today many modern naturopaths consider themselves to be 'natural general practitioners', but their fundamental tenet is that the individual's resistance, will power and determination to overcome disease is paramount. They encourage their patients to eat less refined and more organically grown foods that contain fewer chemicals and pesticides than 'ordinary' foods, so that there is less stress on the organs of excretion such as the liver and kidneys or interference with the body's self-regulatory system. Drugs prescribed by orthodox practitioners are considered to interfere with the healing process and are not used by naturopaths. Sometimes vitamins, tissue salts and other remedies, either homoeopathic or herbal, are prescribed to encourage detoxification and healing of the body.

In the USA naturopaths use many herbal and homoeopathic remedies. In the UK treatment focuses on adjustment to diet, nutritional supplements and herbal medicine. European practitioners use hydrotherapy and herbal medicines. Some practitioners have a specific approach while others draw on a wide range of techniques.

Conditions helped

Naturopathy is particularly helpful for the following problems: acne, addictions, alopecia, anaemia, anorexia nervosa, anxiety, asthma, boils, burns, candidiasis, carpal tunnel syndrome, catarrh, colitis, constipation, cramp, cystitis, dandruff, depression, diverticulitis, eating disorders (compulsive eating, bulimia, anorexia), eczema, excessive sweating, feeling run down, flatulence, fluid retention, gallstones, gout, hay fever, halitosis, headaches (including migraine), haemorrhoids (piles), heavy periods, high blood pressure, high cholesterol levels, hives, hyperactivity, hysteria, impetigo, indigestion, insomnia, irritable bowel syndrome (IBS), kidney stones, leg ulcers, low blood pressure, menstrual problems, migraine, mouth ulcers, myalgic encephalomyelitis (ME), nausea and vomiting in pregnancy or from anaesthesia, night sweats, obesity, osteoarthritis, osteoporosis, painful periods, peptic ulcers, piles, post-natal depression, pre-menstrual syndrome (PMS), psoriasis, Raynaud's disease, sinusitis, sore throats, spots and pimples, stress, tennis elbow, thrush, travel sickness, vaginitis, varicose veins, vertigo and water retention. Naturopathy is also helpful for any chronic condition that conventional medicine has been unable to diagnose or treat.

How to find a therapist

Contact a national naturopathic organization (see Part IV) for details of fully qualified therapists.

What to expect

Naturopaths treat each person as unique. At the first session you will undergo a very thorough physical examination. You may have some blood tests, a urine analysis and possibly X-rays. Your hair may be inspected, together with your nails, skin and mucous membranes of the mouth and tongue, and there will be routine inspection of the heart, pulse, lungs and blood pressure. Your spinal joints and other parts of the musculoskeletal system may be checked. In addition you will be asked questions about your medical history, present state of health and lifestyle. You may be asked how you react to different types of weather, or how you tend to feel at different times of the day. You may also be asked about your eating habits, sleep patterns, menstrual cycles, bowel movements and frequency of urination. Very close attention will be paid to your mental and emotional state as naturopaths think that feelings of hate, self-pity, worry, fear and other negative emotions produce poisonous toxins.

When the underlying cause of the problem has been established a plan of treatment will be drawn up. You will almost certainly be asked to change your diet to ensure that it includes plenty of fruit, a small amount of organic meat and no sugar, refined foods, alcohol, tea or coffee. Tobacco will also have to be eliminated. You may be asked to keep a diary for a few weeks while your practitioner eliminates certain foods to see how your body responds. You may be asked to fast, that is, abstain from eating any food, for two to three days, and only drink water. You may experience a 'healing crisis' after a few weeks of naturopathic treatment, in the form of a cold, cough, fever or loose bowels. This is thought to be a positive response to treatment.

Limitations and dangers

Naturopathy is not suitable for any condition caused by a serious underlying disease, serious infections or a serious psychiatric illness.

Fasting and special diets must be closely monitored and professionally supervised. Note that fasting does *not* cleanse the liver, which is actually overworked because it is flooded with toxins as a result of no food passing through.

Osteopathy

Definition and principles

Osteopathy is a holistic system of diagnosis and treatment that focuses on structural and mechanical problems of the musculoskeletal system of the body. There is special emphasis on the spinal column, muscles, joints and tissues of the periphery. The aim is to correct problems in the body frame, making it easier for the body to function normally and reducing the likelihood of problems occurring in the future.

Brief outline

Andrew Taylor Still was an American doctor, a physician from Missouri who studied engineering. During the 1870s he developed a new system of treatment that emphasized the importance of the spine. Still claimed that as the body had its own healing mechanism, all that was required were adjustments to allow the natural healing process to begin.

Andrew Still believed in two fundamental principles. The first was that structure governs function, and function structure. He maintained structure and function in the human body were completely interdependent; if the structure of the body became altered or abnormal in any way, the body's function would also alter. The second principle was that the role of the artery is supreme. Still claimed that if the arterial blood supply was normal, the bodily structure would function normally, but if it was abnormal the bodily structure would change and disease might occur. He saw the human body fitting together as a jigsaw puzzle and considered it to be naturally healthy with its own healing processes and vital spirit. He believed disease to be caused partly by spinal vertebrae slipping out of position. If the spine's function as a protective channel for nerves were to be impaired the circulation of the blood would be affected and ill health would result. Nerves leaving the spinal column go to all the organs of the body, so that any problem in the nerves or the spine itself would affect the organs concerned. Conversely, if the organ was diseased in any way, this would affect nerve function and might be carried back to the spine. The spine had to be treated by careful manipulation that would unblock the impediment to the blood flow and allow the body to cure itself.

Today, osteopaths continue to adhere to Andrew Still's principles. It is claimed our bodies depend on the operation of a finely tuned, complex system of bones and joints, and that they are controlled and moved by muscles and actuated by nerves. The bones and joints are surrounded by soft tissue containing the fluids of the circulatory system. Changes in the balance of this neuro-musculoskeletal system and its circulatory components may result in restricted flexibility and mobility, disturbance of the blood supply and malfunction of the nervous system and psyche.

Like Andrew Still, modern day osteopaths believe the structure and function of the human body are completely interdependent. The circulation of blood and lymph fluid ensures the well-being of the whole body at a cellular level. A poor arterial blood supply means the cells are deprived of oxygen and nutrients. A poor venous circulation means waste products and carbon dioxide cannot be removed from the cells and toxins build up. Likewise, a poor lymphatic circulation means the body's defence against viruses and bacteria, for example, is impaired. The proper circulation of the blood, both arterial and venous, and the lymph fluids holds the key to health and healing. By gentle manipulation the osteopath balances the circulation of these fluids and thus supports the body's own healing powers. Treatment also helps the lymphatic system to flush away impurities accumulated in the body's tissues.

In the USA osteopathy is now part of orthodox medical practice. Elsewhere, however, this is not the case. In the UK the General Osteopathic Council has a statutory duty to set and enforce standards of professional training and practice, and only registered practitioners are allowed to describe themselves as registered osteopaths: nevertheless, osteopathy is still an alternative therapy. In the UK, as in other English-speaking countries in the West, osteopaths prefer to be called complementary practitioners.

Conditions helped

About 90 per cent of conditions treated by osteopaths are musculoskeletal related conditions, although non-musculoskeletal problems may also be treated. There has been particular success claimed in treating the following conditions: arthritis, asthma, back pain, carpal tunnel syndrome, catarrh, colic, cramp, frozen shoulder, hay fever, headaches, hyperactivity in children, indigestion, insomnia, joint pains, lumbago, menstrual problems, migraine, neuralgia, post-natal depression, postural problems during pregnancy, Raynard's disease, repetitive strain injury (RSI), respiratory problems, sciatica, sinusitis, sports injuries, tennis elbow, tension headaches, tinnitus, vertigo, and whiplash.

How to find a therapist

It is essential to be treated by a fully qualified and experienced osteopath. If you are treated by someone who is unqualified there is a risk you may be harmed. Contact your doctor or one of the national organizations listed in Part IV for a reputable practitioner.

What to expect

The initial session will probably last for up to an hour. The osteopath will take detailed notes of your medical history, previous illnesses, lifestyle, injuries and current treatments for ailments. Under certain circumstances, your osteopath may want you to have orthopaedic, neurological and circulatory examinations, in addition to X-rays, blood tests and urine analyses.

You will undress down to underclothes and your practitioner will watch you standing still, moving about, bending forwards and sideways, and sitting. He or she will assess your posture and underlying skeletal structure, and will examine your body in detail by a method of touch known as palpation. Restricted or excessive movements of the joints will be carefully noted and the soft tissues, muscles, ligaments and connective tissues examined in detail.

Once the necessary examinations have been completed and a diagnosis made, the osteopath will decide whether or not treatment is likely to help your condition and, if so, what sort of treatment would be suitable and safe for you to receive.

THE THERAPIES

If it is agreed that treatment is suitable, you will lie on a table or stand up in a position determined by your practitioner. Osteopaths work with their hands. Several osteopathic techniques may be employed for one condition; there are no standard treatments, and all treatments are designed to suit the patient.

Massaging soft tissue and articulating the joints stretches the ligaments, relaxes taut muscles and improves the circulatory systems. The osteopath monitors the tissue very carefully.

Gentle, repetitive stretching movements improve joint mobility and reduce tension in the surrounding muscles. These may be used to stretch or break down adhesions, stretch shortened ligaments and promote lymphatic movement, to increase movement within the joint itself. This technique also improves blood circulation and fluid drainage.

Muscle energy techniques originated in the USA and are now popular worldwide. Here the joint is contracted until a barrier is felt by the osteopath. The patient is asked to push the joint into the barrier while the osteopath resists. The osteopath subsequently releases the resistance.

The spine or stiff or disfunctioning peripheral joints may be released by putting the joints through very small fast movements in a very controlled manner. This is known as the 'high velocity thrust' technique, which often causes the joints to click or pop. It is usually completely painless but may be daunting because it is an unusual experience. A skilled practitioner will ensure the practice is painless. Often after treatment with this technique there is a great relief from pain in the spine or reduction in muscle tension.

The circulation of cerebral spinal fluid up the spinal column and around the brain forms a rhythmical involuntary movement that is expressed through all tissues of the body. Cranial osteopathy adjusts the skull slightly to ensure the circulation of cerebral spinal fluid is unimpeded and to relax and balance the whole body. The gentle nature of this treatment makes it particularly appropriate for babies who fail to sleep, children with catarrh, constant colds and ear problems, women who have been a long time in labour with forceps deliveries, and older people.

You may need to see your osteopath only once, but it is more likely you will need several treatments for conditions such as low back pain. Chronic conditions may require treatment for many months. A few days afterwards you may feel bruised, but this feeling will pass. If you suffer a severe reaction (though this is very unlikely), you should at once contact your osteopath who will ask you to return as soon as possible so that the treatment may be modified. It is more likely you will find the treatment pleasant and relaxing. Second and subsequent sessions will probably last for 20–30 minutes.

You will be encouraged to be mobile as quickly as possible. A great deal of advice on lifestyle management and exercise will be given, specifically related to your conditions.

Limitations and dangers

Although most medical practitioners accept the viability of osteopathy for treating musculoskeletal problems, they retain some scepticism if it is used to deal with non-musculoskeletal problems such as catarrh. Osteopathy is not recommended for osteoporosis sufferers when bones are brittle and joints are inflamed.

Pilates

Definition and principles

Pilates is a body conditioning programme comprising movements to help increase flexibility, build up strength and tone muscles, without adding bulk. There are eight main principles: relaxation, co-ordination, alignment, concentration, flowing movements, centring, breathing and stamina.

Brief outline

Pilates was developed by a German, Joseph H Pilates (1887–1967), in the early twentieth century. Pilates was born in Germany but moved to the USA as a young man. The Pilates therapy was developed in the USA in the middle decades of the twentieth century.

Conditions helped

Pilates can help people of all ages, with or without a physical disorder, to gain alignment, balance, co-ordination, flexibility, mobility and strength, to eliminate bad postural habits, relieve stress and improve general health. It may also help prevent the onset of brittle bones, relieve back pain and repetitive strain injury (RSI).

The method can safely be used by pregnant women for proper breathing and body alignment, improving concentration, and for recovery of body shape and tone after pregnancy.

How to find a therapist

It is essential to find a recognized Pilates school with fully qualified trainers who have undergone very rigorous training, including seminar training and 600 apprenticeship hours. Contact a national Pilates organization (see Part IV).

What to expect

At the initial session you will be asked about your medical history and present and past physical problems encountered. You will be shown how to perform precise movements and be taught to engage your mind with your body to perform the movements correctly. The focus is on whatever requires correcting, which will probably be the abdomen, lower back and buttocks, and emphasis is on developing deep torso strength and flexibility, known as 'centring' to ensure proper posture and reduced risk of injury.

Sessions include work on the mat and on various pieces of apparatus. The exercises are executed lying down to eliminate gravity and postural problems and on specially designed beds so that parts of the body can be worked on in isolation and posture constantly corrected. For best results you should work out on a regular basis twice a week for up to one-and-a-half hours at a time.

Limitations and dangers

Pilates is not suitable for anyone with an infectious disease. Only learn Pilates with a fully qualified trainer, otherwise you may come to harm.

Polarity therapy

Definition and principles

Polarity therapy is a system based on the human energy biofield. There is an electromagnetic energy pattern with cycles of expansion and contraction. Disease occurs when there are 'blockages' in this energy field arising from unhealthy lifestyles, trauma and self-defeating attitudes. The aim is to release 'blockages' and achieve a balance of the energy currents.

Brief outline

The system was devised by Dr Randolph Stone (1890–1983), an American who incorporated Eastern principles of yoga and Ayurveda with Western theories of osteopathy.

Conditions helped

Polarity therapists claim to be able to treat any condition. They claim particular success with the following: arthritis, backache, carpal tunnel syndrome, cystitis, eating disorders, excessive sweating, gout, haemorrhoids (piles), irritable bowel syndrome (IBS), kidney stones, menopause, migraine, neuralgia, obesity, painful periods, peptic ulcers, pre-menstrual syndrome (PMS), psoriasis, repetitive strain injuries (RSI), sinusitis, sports injuries, stress, toothache and water retention.

How to find a therapist

Contact a national organization (see Part IV). Make sure you choose a fully qualified practitioner who has been trained for at least 18 months part-time.

What to expect

On your initial visit the therapist will take detailed notes of your medical history, allergies and lifestyle. He or she will need to identify your energy state, which can be done, for instance, by dowsing with a pendulum or pulse diagnosis. Once the energy disturbance has been identified, you will probably have some Polarity bodywork. Different types of pressure are applied to the body. This may be, for instance, a light fingertip touch to restore body awareness and balance, or deep manipulation to stimulate or balance the electromagnetic field.

You will probably be asked to change your diet to include plenty of fruit and vegetables, and to practise simple postures. These help maintain muscle tone, strengthen the spine and release toxins.

Limitations and dangers

Polarity therapy may be dangerous if you suffer from the following conditions: deep vein thrombosis, epilepsy, serious psychiatric illness, shingles or varicose veins.

Psychodrama

Definition and principles

Psychodrama is an action-orientated method that uses theatrical techniques in a clinical context to explore the origins of past emotions. With the help of others, individuals act out real or imaginary situations that are causing them distress. Feelings are expressed openly in a safe and supportive group environment.

Brief outline

The therapy was devised in the 1920s by Jacob Moreno (1892–1974), an Austrian psychiatrist who settled in the USA. He found a way to work on both verbal and non-verbal levels to encourage cathartic release.

Conditions helped

Psychodrama reduces inhibitions, releases suppressed emotions, facilitates greater empathy with others and greater ease in adopting new ways of behaviour. Many have benefited from treatment, particularly those who are physically disabled, those with learning difficulties or those who have eating disorders and other addictive problems.

Choosing a therapist

It is essential to find a fully qualified therapist who knows about group dynamics, how to direct individuals, how to cope with strong emotions, whom you can trust and feel comfortable working with. Contact a national organization (see Part IV).

What to expect

There are five main components to a psychodramatic action, known as an enactment.

- *The place.* Known as the psychodramatic stage. It is free from real-life constraints and therefore safe to explore long-buried painful feelings.
- *The protagonist.* The individual working out problems, portraying scenes from a subjective perspective.
- *The director.* The producer and therapist who has overall responsibility for the psychodrama session.
- *The auxiliaries.* The rest of the cast who act out various roles such as mothers, fathers, siblings, kings, queens or inanimate objects.
- *The audience.* People not involved in the psychodramatic action but who may provide important feedback in the sharing period following enactment.

Enactment often provides emotional release and reduces anxiety. Protagonists are often clearer about their own situations and possible solutions and feel less constrained by emotional baggage.

Limitations and dangers

Psychodrama deals with mental problems; it cannot help with physical illness caused by external circumstances, such as a virus.

Qigong

Definition and principles

Qigong, also spelt chi kung, meaning exercises which work with energy, is a meditational exercise technique. A component of Traditional Chinese Medicine (see p. 134), it is designed to encourage the free flow, and harmonize the circulation, of *Qi* (life energy) around organs of the body. It encourages the body's self-healing mechanisms in the event of illness.

Brief outline

The basis of qigong is a series of simple movements, breathing techniques and meditation. It was originally inspired by instinctive movements of wild animals. The art was suppressed for ten years in China during the cultural revolution but enjoyed a revival at the end of the 1970s and now millions of people practise it every day. It was virtually unknown in the West until very recently.

Conditions helped

Qigong is reputed to alleviate asthma, diabetes, heart disease, high blood pressure, irritable bowel syndrome (IBS), migraines musculoskeletal pain, stiffness, stress-related conditions and tumours. It has been shown to enhance health, well-being and emotional stability.

How to find a therapist

Currently there are not very many practitioners in the West. Contact a national organization (see Part IV) for further information.

What to expect

Practitioners teach exercises and breathing and meditation techniques to stimulate *Qi* in the meridians (the channels through the body along which *Qi* flows). The basic postures are easy to learn and suitable for everyone, including older people. The exercises can be performed in any order and to begin with each one should be repeated many times.

Self treatment

Once you have properly mastered qigong techniques, you can practise them yourself, anywhere at any time. They are not difficult to learn but have to be learnt properly. It is also important to learn the philosophy, the meaning, behind the movements.

Limitations and dangers

Do not use qigong if you suffer from a psychotic illness. Most orthodox practitioners are currently dubious of the claims made by practitioners.

Radionics

Definition and principles

With radionics, both diagnosis and healing are conducted at a distance; the patient and practitioner do not meet. Practitioners use healing energy conducted through a special radionic instrument. The principle of this method of healing is based on a universal energy flow that connects all living things. Illness is caused when the energy of the body is in some way out of balance. The aim is to identify and eliminate the root cause of the disease.

Brief outline

Dr Albert Abrams, a North American physician, first discovered radionics principles over 70 years ago. His discoveries were augmented by a UK engineer, George de la Warr, in Oxford in the UK during the 1940s. The therapy is banned in some States in the USA and today the UK is the world centre of radionics.

Conditions helped

Radionics is used for all health problems, treating the physical, emotional and mental states of humans, other animals and even plants. It is quite safe used with other therapies or in conjunction with orthodox medicine. It has helped with terminal illnesses and some patients have said that radionics has helped them to face up to dying.

How to find a therapist

Contact a national radionics organization for a reputable therapist (see Part IV). If there is no national organization contact a 'general' national organization listed at the beginning of Part IV. It is essential to find someone reputable and qualified who has had at least three years' training.

What to expect

You are sent a case history form which you fill in and return, together with a 'witness', usually a drop of blood or snippet of hair which acts as a link between you and the practitioner. The practitioner carries out an analysis, using a radionic diagnostic instrument that measures your 'vibratory patterns', and assesses the levels of health of the major organs as well as the immune, circulatory and nervous systems. Treatments ('corrective energies') will be broadcast in the form of waves, in a similar way to the sound or light of a television screen.

Limitations and dangers

Although radionics is not harmful, the therapy has not been scientifically proven and is therefore not accepted by orthodox medical practitioners.

Reflexology

Definition and principles

Reflexology aims to treat the whole body through massage applied to specific pressure points of both feet. The feet are perceived to be 'mirrors', or reflect the condition, of specific parts of the body, with the left foot representing areas on the left-hand side and the right foot representing areas on the right-hand side of the body. Practitioners believe that 'energy channels' connect the feet with specific parts of the body, and that health problems stem from blockages in these energy channels. The purpose of the massage is to unblock the channels to restart the flow of energy so that natural healing, without the use of surgery or drugs, can occur.

Brief history

Reflexology was known to the indigenous peoples of Africa and America and was also practised in ancient China and Egypt. Early in the twentieth century, Dr William Fitzgerald, an American ear, nose and throat consultant, became interested in the possibility of treating various organs throughout the body through pressure points that were far removed from the organs themselves. He noted that pressure in specific parts of the body might have an anaesthetizing effect on a related area. His theory was based on the body being divided into ten equal, vertical zones, that ended in the fingers and toes. Fitzgerald used his techniques to anaesthetize patients when performing small operations and also to help women in labour. He called his treatment zone therapy.

Fitzgerald's techniques were developed and refined by Eunice Ingham, an American therapist, during the 1930s into reflexology as it is known today. She concentrated on the feet alone and observed that congestion or tension in any part of the foot mirrored congestion or tension in a corresponding part of the body. The therapy is now one of the most popular alternative therapies practised in the West. Many people claim they have benefited from the therapy although practitioners do not know exactly how the treatment works.

There have been very few trials but the little research that has so far been undertaken has produced positive results in favour of reflexology. A study carried out in January 1990 in a Manchester hospital in the UK indicated that the therapy may significantly reduce anxiety levels and stress. Of a total of nine older patients, three received reflexology treatment, three counselling and three no treatment other than the standard nursing care available, for eight days consecutively. Subsequently, those who had received reflexology treatment showed a marked decrease in anxiety, while the decrease was much less significant in those who had received counselling. Those who had had no treatment reported no change. A US study in 1993 showed that women who suffered severe pre-menstrual syndrome (PMS) and who had reflexology treatments suffered fewer symptoms than a control group who were given placebos over a two-month period.

Conditions helped

Reflexology can be used to alleviate a very wide range of conditions, including the following: acne, addictions, agoraphobia, arthritis, asthma, back pain, breathing disorders, bronchitis, catarrh, circulatory problems, claustrophobia, constipation, cystitis, depression, diarrhoea, ear, nose and throat conditions, eczema, hay fever, heavy periods, indigestion, high blood pressure, hormonal imbalances, incontinence, insomnia, joint problems, kidney disorders, loss of libido, lumbago, menopausal symptoms, menstrual problems, migraine, myalgic encephalomyelitis (ME), neck pain, pre-menstrual syndrome (PMS), post-natal depression, psoriasis, rheumatism, sinusitis, stiffness, stress and tension. Although no reflexologist would ever claim to cure conditions, in fact conditions can often be cleared.

Choosing a therapist

It is extremely important to find a fully qualified and reputable therapist. Unfortunately this may prove difficult. There are very many reflexology organizations partly because the therapy is unregulated. It is best to contact one of the national organizations listed in Part IV.

What to expect

At the initial session the reflexologist will take detailed notes of your medical history and will want to know about the symptoms of any current problems. You will be asked about your lifestyle and diet, which you may be asked to modify.

You will probably be asked to wash and dry your feet and then to sit in a reclining chair, massage couch or an ordinary chair with a foot rest. You will sit with the legs raised, without shoes or socks. The practitioner will first carefully examine your feet, looking for any signs of infection or the presence or absence of hard skin, the state of the nails, any swelling, the temperature and colour of the feet, etc. Talcum powder will be applied to the feet before massage. Both feet will then be given a very thorough massage. The practitioner will use the side of the thumb pressed firmly on to a particular reflex point. The thumb is always kept bent and pressure is released when the thumb is pulled back with a slight circular movement. Sometimes the practitioner's fingers are also used. The massage has to be very precise because each reflex is very small, only about the size of a pin head. The reflexologist will move from one reflex in the foot to another with a forward creeping movement. This is so the thumbs are kept in contact with the foot as much as possible.

There are reflexes in the feet for all parts of the body. They are found mainly on the soles of the feet, but also on the top and sides. The big toes represent the head and the brain; the little toes the sinuses. If specific areas of each foot are massaged, other areas of the body can be affected that are distant to the part of the foot being massaged. By working on the reflexes, the circulation of blood to the corresponding part of the body is improved and a reduction in nervous tension in the area occurs. Reflexology can stimulate the healing forces present in the body and thus increase the body's ability to heal itself.

If the area being worked on is out of balance, a pain will be felt in the foot as pressure is applied. This may be very sharp, rather like a fingernail piercing the skin. Tender areas indicating an imbalance will be given extra massage. This will lessen the pain which should completely disappear after a few minutes. Sometimes small granules can be felt under the skin of the feet which will be dispersed by massage. The residue will be absorbed by the circulatory system and eventually excreted from the body. With every treatment, all areas of the feet are massaged so the body is treated as a whole.

A treatment session usually lasts for about three-quarters of an hour, and you are advised to have at least six to eight treatments. You may find an improvement in your condition after the first session. If there is no change after three sessions, reflexology is probably not the right treatment for your current problem.

Following treatment, you may experience a number of reactions. You may feel quite tired; your sleep patterns may change; you may sweat more; if you are a woman you may have increased vaginal discharge; you may need to urinate or defecate more frequently; you may develop a slight skin rash, a sore throat or a runny nose. Reflexologists believe that these reactions, all of which are quite common, are because the body is striving to release toxins. Any unpleasant reaction will normally only be present for up to 48 hours. You will also probably experience a significant reduction in stress, even after the first session. You may also feel revitalized, rather than tired, and experience a sense of well-being.

It is suggested that reflexology treatment at regular intervals can help to maintain the body in a healthy state.

Self treatment

Only very minor ailments are suitable for self-treatment and you should ask your practitioner what techniques to use and be shown how to perform them. If, as is very probable, you find it awkward to work on your own feet, you can work on corresponding reflex areas in the hands instead. Never try to work from reading texts or looking at illustrations in books. However much information is provided, it is quite impossible to show the precise parts of the feet that require massage. If you do try to work on yourself without the help of a practitioner, you will almost certainly gain no benefit.

Limitations and dangers

Reflexology often has powerful effects on the body. You should not have reflexology treatment if you have phlebitis (inflammation of a vein) or thrombosis (blood clotting). The following conditions can be treated but great care must be taken, and in some instances treatment may not be appropriate: arthritis in the feet, diabetes, any thyroid disorder, osteoporosis, heart trouble or shingles. It is suggested you do not have treatment if you are pregnant or on high dose drugs. Also, reflexology is not suitable for any condition that may be caused by serious underlying disease.

Reiki

Definition and principles

Reiki is a hands-on healing system for channelling the life force. The name derives from two Japanese words: *rei*, meaning universal and spiritual, and *ki* (*Qi*), life force energy. The therapy works on all levels: spiritual, mental, emotional and physical. The practitioner acts as a channel for healing energy.

Brief outline

The therapy was developed out of ancient Tibetan Buddhist healing practices by Dr Mikao Usi, a Japanese theologian in the late nineteenth century. It was brought to the West in the mid 1960s by a Japanese woman, Hawaio Takata.

The most noticeable effect after treatment is elimination of stress and a feeling of relaxation and well-being.

Conditions helped

Reiki is suitable for people of any age, and is particularly effective for relieving stress-related conditions such as headaches, insomnia and general anxiety.

How to find a therapist

Choose a reputable therapist, that is, one who has been given training by a Reiki Master. The Reiki Alliance with addresses in the USA and Europe (see Part IV) has up-to-date information about practitioners worldwide.

What to expect

A practitioner will take a detailed history of your problems and lifestyle. You lie down on your back while the practitioner places hands over a number of strategic places on your body. You may feel energy flow into these places in the form of heat, cold or a tingling sensation. Most treatments last for at least an hour, sometimes considerably longer.

Self treatment

You can treat yourself using Reiki techniques, and patients are encouraged to do so, as the more one takes charge of oneself the more likely one is to heal. Initial training is, however, essential. There are three levels of qualifications ('degrees'), and to self-treat you must train to at least the first degree level. Self treatment involves meditation and scanning the body to find areas that need 'retuning'.

Limitations and dangers

Reiki is not recommended for treating chronic or acute conditions.

Rolfing

Definitions and principles

Rolfing, a method of structural integration, uses deep tissue massage that manipulates fascia – the thin, elastic connective tissue (see p. 74). This eases back, neck and joint pain and helps to resolve emotional issues shown in body posture and movements.

Brief history

Rolfing was created in the 1930s by Ida Rolf, an American biochemist. It is a system of firm pressure and manipulation designed to bring the whole body into correct vertical alignment. Dr Rolf believed the body has a natural symmetry, enabling it to work in harmony with gravity, but that injury, poor posture or emotional distress can throw it out of alignment.

Conditions helped

Rolfing alleviates anxiety, back and neck pain, painful periods, stiff or painful joints and chronic structural imbalance. It also prevents postural or stress-related problems. The therapy is used by dancers, musicians and sports people to ensure their bodies are in optimum condition.

THE THERAPIES

Choosing a therapist

There are few practitioners: in 1998 there were only about 700 worldwide. If there is no rolfing organization in your country, contact the headquarters in the USA (see Part IV).

What to expect

Deep massage and pressure are applied to specific areas of the body with fingers, hands, elbows and knees. This may be painful, but only very briefly. You are asked to breathe and move in certain ways to help the practitioner. There is a set course of ten weekly treatments, with each session focusing on specific areas of the body. The final three or four sessions are used to 'reset' muscles and fine-tune posture.

After a session you will almost certainly feel lighter and walk taller. You may feel a bit sore for a few days and experience an emotional release from tension.

Limitations and dangers

Avoid rolfing if you are pregnant, if you have any infectious disease, deep vein thrombosis, shingles, or have scar tissue or varicose veins. Rolfing is not suitable for people who bruise easily or who are obese. The therapy it does not claim to cure disease.

Shiatsu

Definition and principles

Shiatsu, meaning 'finger pressure', is a Japanese massage technique based on the principles of Traditional Chinese Medicine (TCM) (see pp. 134–7). The treatment encourages a steady flow of Qi, correcting imbalances so that overall health is increased and many health problems alleviated.

Brief outline

Shiatsu was developed early in the twentieth century in Japan. It became widely known in the West in the 1970s.

Conditions helped

Shiatsu helps to alleviate many conditions including: arthritis, asthma, circulation problems, digestive disorders, headaches, insomnia, menstrual problems, musculoskeletal problems, stress and tiredness. The technique promotes deep relaxation and is claimed to regulate the hormonal system and the circulation of blood and lymphatic fluids. Regular shiatsu sessions help prevent illness. Treatment enhances digestion and alleviates circulatory problems. It aids emotional stability and helps to promote self-confidence and peace of mind.

How to find a therapist

It is essential to find a reputable therapist. Contact a national organization (see Part IV).

What to expect

At the initial session you will be diagnosed according to the 'four examinations' system of TCM. You do not have to undress for treatment but should wear a single layer of cotton garments. You lie on a mat or on the floor while you receive treatment. Each session covers the whole body. To begin with, the palms and fingertips will be used to feel for problem areas in your body. Thumbs and fingertips are used if specific pressure has to be applied to a pressure point, known as a *tsubos* or acupoint, otherwise the palms of the hands tend to be used. If very strong pressure is needed, the elbows, feet and knees may be used. Each session lasts for about an hour.

Limitations and dangers

Shiatsu is not suitable if you have the following conditions: epilepsy, high blood pressure, osteoporosis, thrombosis or varicose veins. It is best to avoid shiatsu if you are pregnant. Do not eat or take strenuous exercise for an hour before or after shiatsu treatment.

Sound therapy

Definition and principles

Sound therapy is based on the principle that the organs and cells of the body resonate at particular sound frequencies. Illness affects the resonance and changes the frequencies.

Brief outline

Therapists enable a patient's voice and electronic or musical instruments to generate sound waves that restore balance and promote healing.

Conditions helped

The therapy is used to help children with behavioural problems and learning difficulties. It is useful for those who suffer from headaches, gout, high blood pressure, stress, tension and depression. It is also used to treat muscle and joint pains, arthritis and rheumatic complaints, and has proved effective after bone surgery to speed recovery.

How to find a therapist

Contact a national organization (see Part IV) for a fully qualified practitioner.

What to expect

A sound therapist will first take a detailed history of your past and present illnesses and will analyse your voice to make a prognosis. A fearful voice, for example, indicates a bladder problem. If it sounds angry, this may throw light on a liver or gall-bladder disease. Once the problem is diagnosed you may be given chants or mantras to sing in various notes. Using your voice in a certain way, together with rhythmic breathing music, can help you to relax, heighten awareness and change electrical brainwave patterns. Harmonious sound waves can be directed at problem areas of the body and help to regenerate balance. You may be asked to listen to sounds and music and perform frequent voice and physical exercises to loosen up the body.

Other sound therapies, such as Cymatic therapy, use high frequency sound waves (ultrasound) to stimulate the body to heal itself.

Limitations and dangers

The therapy may exacerbate psychotic behaviour such as schizophrenia.

T'ai chi ch'uan

Definition and principles

T'ai chi ch'uan, usually shortened to t'ai chi, is a Chinese martial art. It was originally employed for the purpose of self defence but is now used for health and spiritual development by encouraging Qi, (life energy). T'ai chi is also used as a therapy for the prevention and treatment of disease. You learn how to think and move in ways governed by principles and methods of practice. You are taught to become aware of the natural laws that govern change and are encouraged to think about the mechanisms of change and movements that govern all aspects of our lives and the world about us.

Brief outline

T'ai chi was originally devised as a martial art by Taoist monks in China during the Yuan dynasty (1271–1368). Later, however, as the exercises were seen to benefit people's health, they were used both to prevent and treat disease. Today in China, t'ai chi is used in hospitals for the treatment of chronic disease and people are encouraged to exercise every day to keep in good health and prevent disease. In the parks in China people are seen exercising up to a very advanced age.

There are six main t'ai chi principles, rooted in Traditional Chinese Medicine (TCM) (see pp. 134–7). Some are quite difficult to understand unless you have had first-hand experience of the exercises, but if you practise t'ai chi they will gradually begin to make sense and become very much part of your life. You are taught to relax both your mind and body, in order to discover your inner strength and become centred and focused. You are also shown how important it is to concentrate, to keep the mind connected to what your body is experiencing. You are taught how to enable the body and mind to respond spontaneously to immediate needs of the moment. Through the exercises you are shown how to be consistent in your thoughts and actions, so that you can achieve your goals. You are also taught to value slow but steady progress and, if necessary, to delay the gratification of achievement, to allow time to gain what you want. The final principle, which perhaps is the most difficult to achieve, is to learn to accept life's challenges.

Conditions helped

In the West, t'ai chi is increasingly recognized by orthodox practitioners as having therapeutic potential and currently is used for combating stress and stress-related problems. It has also proved to help people to recover from physical injuries and to aid cardiac rehabilitation. T'ai chi can help people to relax, acting as an alternative to tranquillizers, and prevent anxiety and stress. It also helps with breathing problems and stimulates the circulation, tones up body muscles and improves posture. T'ai chi can not only reduce both verbal and physical aggression but, if properly practised, can also channel aggression into more positive action. It is particularly suitable and valuable for older people because it is a gentle, measured form of exercise, helping not only to increase balance and muscle strength but also to reduce arthritis. During recent years, an increasing number of athletes have taken up t'ai chi to keep fit and help them concentrate on their sports.

How to find a teacher

A skilful t'ai chi teacher is essential. Choose one who has had at least four years' experience from a reputable training establishment (see Part IV).

What to expect

For the exercises you will need to wear comfortable, loose-fitting clothes. You will learn many movements, a lot of which are circular, that are linked together in a continuous stream. These are practised slowly and smoothly, in a clearly defined pattern, co-ordinated with regular breathing and with precise postural alignment. You will also learn how to concentrate the mind and to become focused. For the exercises to be effective, as benefits are gained only gradually, you need to practise for at least 90 minutes per week. Although the work you will be doing is not physically strenuous, it is nevertheless complex, and requires a lot of physical and, particularly, mental effort. You will be told you should move like a cat that feels the ground before it puts its paws down and that your level of attentiveness should be as great as that of a cat about to pounce on a mouse. You will need patience to persevere and learn how to adapt and change both your physical movements and thoughts and attitudes relating to your goals and what goes on in your life.

There are two types of t'ai chi in the West. The short form consists of 40 to 60 movements conducted over a period of five to ten minutes. The long form involves more than 100 movements, with an exercise period lasting from 20 to 40 minutes. This includes repetitions that are considered essential to achieve physical and psychological balance. The two forms of the exercise both concentrate more on mental rather than physical attributes, as it is considered crucial to strengthen concentration and to become focused. Health is considered to be natural and effortless for an individual who has achieved balance and harmony between body and mind.

You need to repeat and refine constantly what you have been taught. As well as improving posture and balance, daily practice focuses the mind, calms emotions and relaxes the body. A good student will gradually become well grounded, confident and at ease with the world.

Limitations and dangers

It is essential to learn t'ai chi from a skilled teacher, and it will take at least six months to master the exercises. There will come a time, however, when you will have learnt the techniques sufficiently to be able to practise on your own. You must learn the art of t'ai chi properly. As long as you have done this there are no known adverse side-effects. If you have not been properly taught and have not learnt how to move or think according to t'ai chi principles, you may well experience problems.

Traditional Chinese Medicine

Definition and principles

In *Chung-i* (Traditional Chinese Medicine – TCM), both health and illness have physical, emotional and spiritual dimensions. The emphasis is on preventing disease and recognizing symptoms of pre-disease. It is said the body is naturally disposed to gravitate towards *tao* (equilibrium), the absolute way of nature, the primeval law that regulates all heavenly and earthly matters.

THE THERAPIES

The principles of TCM are very different from those of Western orthodox medicine. They require a different way of thinking about disease and also life and the way it is, and should, be lived.

Allopathic medicine tends to treat disease symptoms as they arise. They are isolated and controlled or destroyed with drugs or surgery. It describes many physiological processes in great detail but says nothing about the life force or why healing responses vary from person to person. TCM, however, adopts an holistic approach to medicine. Each individual is seen as a unique and integrated combination of mind, body and spirit. The practitioner does take disease symptoms into account, but also age, personal habits and physical and emotional traits, to evaluate patterns of disharmony that have arisen and to assess the type and length of treatment required. The disease symptoms are considered to be merely a part of the disharmony.

Qi (or *Chi*), like *prana* in Indian philosophy, is an invisible life energy that activates all life. In an individual it is the vital energy of the person that circulates around the body. Dual flows of energy, known as *yin* and *yang*, are contained within the *Qi* that are both opposing and complementary forces in nature. They are primordial energies that regulate the universe. Yin cannot exist without yang or yang without yin, and each is constantly changing into its converse. Yang energy is incipient. It sets something in motion, it is something moving or transforming and it communicates motion. It develops, expands, dissolves and disperses. It is indeterminate yet determining. Yin energy completes, confirms, responds, reposes. It is quiescent, static, sustaining, conserving, preserving, condensing and closes in. It is awaiting organization yet is determinate.

Health is maintained as long as *Qi* flows freely through the *Jing* (meridians or channels in the body) and yin and yang are in equilibrium. There are 12 main channels, six yin and six yang, connected with various parts of the body. These comprise a network of invisible pathways in the body. The channels can become blocked, which causes the dynamic of yin and yang in the body to be disturbed. If yang is in excess, the body will be hot. There may be a fever, a dry mouth, the person may be angry or tense. If yin is in excess, the body will be cold and the person will catch colds easily. TCM aims to remove obstructions and allow the *Qi* to flow freely. The symptoms are never treated in isolation from the whole organism.

A second tradition of TCM is known as the five transitional phases, or more popularly as the five elements. The elements are fire, water, earth, metal and wood. Each is associated with both yin and yang organs and specific seasons, tastes and emotions.

- Fire is associated with summer, bitter taste, joy, laughter, manic depression, the heart, small intestine, tongue, blood vessels, sweat, the colour red and the south.
- Earth is associated with late summer, sweet taste, saliva, obsession, worry, sympathy, the spleen, stomach, the singing voice, mouth and muscles, the colour yellow and the centre.
- Metal is associated with autumn, pungent taste, anguish, weeping, the lungs, large intestine, nose, the sense of smell, skin, body hair, the colour white and the west.
- Water is associated with winter, salty taste, fear, the kidneys, bladder, ears, hair, bones, hearing, urine, groaning, the colour black and the north.
- Wood is associated with spring, sour taste, anger, the liver, gall-bladder, tendons, eyes, muscles, tears, depression, shouting, the colour green and the east.

One element can inhibit or support another's function. For instance water (kidneys – yin) inhibits (extinguishes) fire. Fire (heart – yang) inhibits (melts) metal. Metal (lungs – yin) inhibits (cuts) wood. Wood (liver – yin) inhibits (breaks through) earth. Earth (spleen – yin) inhibits (absorbs) water. Conversely, metal (lungs – yin) creates (liquefies) water. Water (kidneys – yin) creates wood. Wood (liver – yin) creates (fuels) fire. Fire (heart – yang) creates (turns to ashes) earth. Earth (spleen – yin) creates (finds underground) metal.

A third tradition is that of the eight principles. These are four pairs of opposites: yin-yang, interior-exterior, cold-hot and empty-full. The first named of the pairs are yin and the second yang (thus, interior – yin, exterior – yang; cold – yin, hot – yang; etc). The eight principles form the eight principal patterns of potential disharmony. All known diseases can be grouped within this framework. Thus, if an individual is diagnosed as too cold, hot treatment will be applied; if too yin, yang treatment will then be administered (although there may be 'false cold', that is, there are some fevers where heat will aggravate the condition and cold needs to be applied).

THE THERAPIES

TCM can treat any illness. The following therapies are based on TCM principles: acupressure (see p. 27), acupuncture (see p. 28), Chinese herbal medicine (see p. 75), kinesiology (see p. 95); qigong (see p. 120), shiatsu (see p. 129) and t'ai chi (see p. 132). Each therapy has a list of conditions it can treat.

Western orthodox medicine entered China at the end of the seventeenth century and by the late nineteenth century threatened to override TCM. The Communist Party was originally committed to the latter's final eradication, but after the People's Republic was established in 1949 both medical systems were allowed to continue in tandem. Today, TCM is practised alongside Western medicine in all hospitals in China. During the past 20 years its popularity has rapidly grown in the West, particularly in countries with large Chinese populations, for example, Australia, the UK and USA.

How to find a therapist

If you are seeking a TCM therapist you need to choose one of the specialist therapies listed above, each with its own method of treatment. If in doubt about which to choose, contact a national TCM organization (see Part IV).

Limitations and dangers

TCM is based on very different premises to that of allopathic medicine and is thus regarded with great suspicion by most Westerners. More familiarity with TCM principles may lead to greater acceptance by orthodox practitioners, but it may be impossible to prove the validity of many of the therapies because they are not based on scientific principles.

Trager bodywork

Definition and principles

Trager bodywork promotes physical mobility, deep relaxation and greater self-awareness and aims to break down neuromuscular patterns such as bad posture, inefficient movement, stiffness and tension. Practitioners use gentle, rhythmic non-intrusive movements such as rocking, cradling and stretching so that the patient is never in pain. The movements help the body to enter a state of profound relaxation.

Brief outline

Trager bodywork was developed by Dr Milton Trager (1908–97). He started out in the 1920s as a professional boxer but gave up this profession after a bodywork session he performed on his trainer, who was immediately convinced Trager had a special gift with his hands. To preserve his hands Trager then worked as an acrobat and dancer. At the same time he relieved his father's sciatic pain and subsequently helped people with polio, spasticity and other physical conditions. After the Second World War he trained as a medical doctor, setting up a private medical practice in Hawaii and working in obscurity. He continued to use his hands and develop his bodywork techniques. He eventually settled in California in 1980 and founded the Trager Institute, training others to use his specialized techniques. There are now (1999) around 2000 Trager bodywork practitioners worldwide.

There are no techniques in Trager bodywork and no claims to produce specific results. Trager is not a medical treatment. Rather, it is an approach, a way of learning and of teaching movement re-education. The aim is to promote feelings of lightness, freedom and well-being.

Conditions helped

Practitioners of Trager bodywork have claimed that the following conditions have been alleviated with treatment: aches, asthma, depression, high blood pressure, migraine, neuromuscular conditions, pain, poor posture, sciatica, stress-related conditions and tension. It is also claimed that the therapy can alleviate some of the symptoms of Parkinson's disease.

How to find a therapist

If you can, contact a national organization for further information. If none is listed, contact one of the 'general' alternative organizations listed at the beginning of Part IV. It is essential to find a qualified Trager bodywork practitioner. You may be harmed if you receive treatment from someone who is not qualified.

What to expect

At the initial session you will be assessed by the Trager bodywork practitioner and will be given a thorough physical examination. You will be asked to undress to your underwear and will then be cradled, stretched or rocked (no massage is involved). The practitioner will be in a state of relaxed, active meditation known as 'hook up'. This state will allow him or her to sense areas of tension in your body and to be constantly aware of your responses. You will be asked to feel a sense of freedom and weightlessness in those areas and be encouraged to let go of your muscular control. You will learn to recognize and let go of unconscious holding patterns, both physical and emotional. This will help to reduce stress, friction and tension. Resilience and mobility will be increased by the elimination of poor patterns of movement and poor self-image. The bodywork will support and expand your desired self-expression and enhance a conscious awareness of the holistic integration of body, mind and spirit. At the same time it can activate feelings of peace, security and a state of well-being.

After treatment you may feel much lighter and free from pain. You may need only one session but it is more likely you will require several treatments. Each session will last for up to one-and-a-half hours.

Self treatment

You will be given a programme of gentle self-treatment known as *Mentastics*, a word coined by Dr Trager and his wife meaning 'mental gymnastics' a series of dance-like movements. This is to help maintain the positive feelings and well-being obtained in Trager bodywork sessions with your practitioner. The aim is to restore and maintain agelessness of body and mind.

Limitations and dangers

Trager bodywork is not recommended for those suffering from osteoporosis or thrombosis. Most orthodox practitioners are sceptical about benefits claimed by practitioners.

Visualization

Definition and principles

Visualization is similar to dreaming. It is a conscious attempt to imagine positive images to benefit health and well-being, create healing and to reinforce positive feelings, behaviour and self image. Visualization therapists believe the mind and body are bound together, so that emotions, images and sensations are linked with the physical body.

Brief outline

For thousands of years, shamans, witch doctors and priests have conjured up images for healing. Today, visualization is used by doctors to help heal many physical and emotional problems.

Conditions helped

Visualization is used to help breathing and relaxation and to alleviate allergies, anxiety, auto-immune diseases, heart conditions, phobias and stress-related conditions. Using the technique improves motivation and changes negative attitudes. It has helped older people create a more positive image of old age for themselves and a greater resistance to illness.

How to find a therapist

It is difficult to find a therapist who is qualified only in visualization techniques. Look for therapists who practise the technique in related fields such as biofeedback or autogenic training (see Part IV).

What to expect

Once your problem has been diagnosed the visualization therapist will ask you to imagine a scene related to your problem. You can draw on any images, for example, people, works of art or landscapes. You talk about the images and try to feel physical and emotional sensations related to them. Your therapist will help you to create adjustments so that negative aspects of the images you perceive give way to positive ones. This is known as 'guided imagery'. Imagining positive images and desired outcomes to specific situations will help you overcome both emotional and physical problems. It is important to note that in visualization you are in a deeply relaxed state but not hypnotized.

Self treatment

It is essential to learn visualization techniques from a qualified practitioner, but once learned the technique may be practised at home.

Limitations and dangers

With serious conditions, visualization should always be used in conjunction with other treatments.

Yoga

Definitions and principles

The word 'yoga' derives from a word in Sanskrit meaning 'union' or 'yoke'. It is a method of training the body, mind and spirit.

Brief outline

Yoga is an extremely ancient practice and existed in India at least 4,000 years ago. It was originally known only to a small élite who abandoned worldly ways for mystical practices and who lived apart in forests or caves. Those who were teachers of the discipline worked out some of the yogic postures by watching and imitating the movements of wild animals.

There are many different kinds of yoga. The method that has been taken up in the West is hatha yoga, from the Sanskrit 'ha' meaning 'sun' and 'tha', 'moon', implying balance. Hatha yoga is the physical expression of yogic practices demonstrated through physical postures. It is a holistic approach to self-development and a means of self-help towards physical and mental health.

Many orthodox practitioners as well as alternative therapists are becoming increasingly interested in yoga with its emphasis on awareness and control of both body and mind. Recently there has been a great deal of research into yoga with much positive feedback. For example, in 1983 the UK Yoga Biomedical Trust investigated the reactions of 2,700 people who practised yoga and were suffering from one or more of 20 different problems. For each condition, over 70 per cent of the people claimed that yoga had helped their condition to improve. Out of a total figure of 1,142 suffering from back pain, 98 per cent said their back pain had been alleviated, and of 834 people suffering from anxiety symptoms, 94 per cent said their symptoms had been alleviated by practising yoga. Another British study in 1994 indicated that yoga could benefit people with rheumatoid arthritis.

Conditions helped

The aim of therapeutic yoga traditionally has been to promote and maintain a healthy mind and body, although recently it has increasingly been used to treat symptoms of disease. It has helped to alleviate the following conditions: addictions, anorexia nervosa, anxiety, arthritis, asthma, breathing problems, bronchitis, bulimia nervosa, circulation problems, constipation, depression, digestive disorders, fatigue, headaches, high blood pressure, hives, hyperventilation, lumbago, menopausal problems, menstrual problems, migraines, psoriasis, rheumatoid arthritis, stress and tension. Additionally, yoga helps people to relax and is instrumental in providing greater strength, suppleness and better posture.

How to find a therapist

It is very important to find a reputable and fully qualified yoga teacher. Contact a national organization (see Part IV).

What to expect

Wear comfortable clothing that stretches and work barefoot on a mat on the floor.

There are no set patterns of teaching hatha yoga. Ideally a yoga teacher should tailor routines to suit each individual. The aim is to integrate the mind and body. Physical postures known as *asanas* may be performed by either standing, kneeling, sitting or lying on your back or front. Each asana should be performed slowly and deliberately, working on both sides of the body. The postures should be held for at least a minute or more to build up awareness of your body, its tensions and patterns of behaviour. Don't try to rush the exercises. There should be no strain involved. Remember that you are not in competition with anyone. As each asana has its own unique shape it is important to maintain each correctly and to practise regularly. Most asanas work on the spine to keep it supple. You may find you experience some stiffness of the joints when you start to practise yoga but if you learn the techniques properly you should never have severe pain.

There are regular intervals when deep relaxation exercises are taught as well as controlled breathing exercises known as *pranayama*. You will probably be taught the basic philosophy of yoga, which includes learning about the 'eight limbs' of yoga, that is: *yamas* (restraints), *niyamas* (observances), *asana* (posture), *pranayama* (breathing control), *pratyahara* (sense withdrawal), *dharana* (concentration), *dhyana* (meditation), and *samadhi* (heightened awareness). The eight limbs are considered essential to the yoga way of life and death.

Each session with a practitioner will last for up to an hour-and-a-half to two hours.

Self treatment

You are advised to learn all yoga techniques, even the most simple ones, from an experienced practitioner. It is essential to perform the asanas correctly. If you don't you will gain no benefit and some of the exercises may be unnecessarily painful. Practise the techniques you have been taught for about half an hour each day. It is very important to progress slowly at a steady pace and not to force yourself. Have a bath or shower after you have completed the exercises to ensure your body and mind are relaxed and try to rest for about half an hour afterwards.

Regular daily practice will provide many benefits such as enhanced concentration, increased energy and stamina and toned-up muscles. It can also help you deal with stress, improve your digestion and, most important of all, give you the feeling that you can cope with all that life deals, that you are in control.

Limitations and dangers

It is important to bear the following points in mind when practising yoga techniques.

- Make sure you learn the techniques with a reputable, fully qualified and experienced yoga teacher.
- Allow at least three hours after a meal before practising any yoga technique.
- Many asanas are dangerous if you are suffering from the following conditions: back or neck injuries, brain disorders, circulation problems, detached retina, heart disease or high blood pressure. Always check each exercise with your yoga teacher and act on the advice given to you, especially if you are pregnant.
- If you are pregnant there are a number of asanas that are unsuitable. Check with your practitioner.

- If you are menstruating there are a number of asanas that are unsuitable. Check with your practitioner.
- Don't practise yoga techniques with either a full bladder or full bowels. If you do you may harm yourself.
- Don't practise yoga techniques immediately after you have taken strenuous exercise.
- Don't practise yoga if you have previously been exposed to strong sunlight.
- Consult your doctor before taking up yoga if you are taking any form of medication or have some form of physical disability.
- There are a number of conditions such as diabetes, Menières disease, MS and ME where you will need a specialist yoga remedial teacher.

Part III
LIST OF PROBLEMS AND THERAPIES FOR TREATMENT

Below are listed over 100 common problems, their symptoms and a choice of up to four alternative therapies that have proved suitable for treatment for each problem. The problems have been given their common names and sometimes have their medical names in brackets if these are well known. They have been given the symptoms that orthodox practitioners consider to be commonly associated with them. Note, however, that some alternative therapies, particularly Eastern medicines such as Ayurveda and Traditional Chinese Medicine (TCM), would describe both the symptoms and problems very differently.

Name of problem	Symptoms	Alternative therapies
abscess	pus in skin tissue	Ayurveda, Chinese herbal medicine, homoeopathy
acne	pimples, blackheads, oily skin	aromatherapy, auto-suggestion, dance therapy, naturopathy
agoraphobia	fear of open spaces, cannot leave familiar setting	art therapy, biofeedback, breathing and relaxation
alcoholism	dependence on alcohol, loss of memory, judgement	acupuncture, biofeedback, meditation, naturopathy
amnesia	partial or total loss of memory	Bach flower remedies, visualization
anaemia	great tiredness, pallor, poor resistance to infection	acupuncture, aromatherapy, homoeopathy, naturopathy
anorexia nervosa	self-induced severe loss of weight	art therapy, massage, naturopathy, psychodrama
anxiety	diarrhoea, sleeplessness, breathlessness	acupuncture, aromatherapy, psychodrama, reiki
arthritis	swelling of joints, pain, restricted motion, red skin	naturopathy, shiatsu Western herbal medicine
asthma	wheezing, difficulty with breathing	acupuncture, Buteyko method, colour therapy, reflexology
athlete's foot	itching between the toes	aromatherapy, Western herbal medicine
back pain	restricted joint movement, pain, nerve pressure	acupuncture, Alexander Technique, chiropractic
bad breath (halitosis)	smell of bad breath	homoeopathy, naturopathy, Western herbal medicine

ALTERNATIVE MEDICINE

baldness (alopecia)	absence of hair on head	aromatherapy, homoeopathy, naturopathy
bedwetting (enuresis)	involuntary urination when asleep at night	aromatherapy, chiropractic, cranial osteopathy
Bell's palsy	paralysis of facial nerve, inability to close an eye	acupuncture, homoeopathy, massage, naturopathy
bleeding gums (gingivitis)	inflammation of gums that are swollen and bleeding	Ayurveda, homoeopathy, naturopathy, Western herbal medicine
blisters	swelling of skin filled with fluid. Sometimes blood, pus	aromatherapy, Western herbal medicine
boils	inflamed area of skin containing pus	Ayurveda, Chinese herbal medicine, naturopathy
bronchitis	inflammation of bronchi, air passages behind windpipe	acupuncture, aromatherapy, Western herbal medicine
bruises (contusions)	skin discoloration	aromatherapy, homoeopathy, Western herbal medicine
bulimia nervosa	excess overeating, leading to vomiting	acupuncture, aromatherapy, hypnotherapy, psychodrama
burns	swelling, blistering of skin, perhaps infection	hydrotherapy, naturopathy, Western herbal medicine
bursitis	inflammation of bursas, small sacs that lubricate the joints	acupuncture, aromatherapy, hydrotherapy, massage
candidiasis	infection in moist areas of body, e.g. mouth and vagina	Ayurveda, hydrotherapy, naturopathy
carpal tunnel syndrome	numbness, pins and needles in fingers, thumb weakness	acupuncture, acupressure, chiropractic, naturopathy
catarrh	secretion of thick phlegm through nose or mouth	acupressure, aromatherapy, hydrotherapy, naturopathy
chilblains	itchy red swelling of skin on extremities (fingers/toes)	acupressure, hydrotherapy, massage, naturopathy
claustrophobia	fear of enclosed, confined places, e.g. lifts, tunnels	art therapy, biofeedback, breathing and relaxation

LIST OF PROBLEMS AND THERAPIES FOR TREATMENT

cold sores (herpes simplex)	inflamed small blisters on the skin	acupuncture, aromatherapy, naturopathy
common cold	inflamed mucous membranes of nose and throat	aromatherapy, Chinese and Western herbal medicine
colic	severe spasmodic abdominal pain	acupressure, cranial osteopathy
conjunctivitis (pink eye)	red, swollen eyes with discharge	Chinese and Western herbal medicine, homoeopathy
constipation	very infrequent elimination of faeces	acupressure, Ayurveda, massage, naturopathy
cramp	spasm of muscles	acupressure, homoeopathy, massage, yoga
croup	inflammation of larynx, difficult breathing	aromatherapy, homoeopathy
cystitis	burning sensation when urinating	acupressure, homoeopathy, naturopathy, Western herbal medicine
dandruff (scurf)	flaky, scaly dead skin on scalp and eyebrows	aromatherapy, homoeopathy, massage, naturopathy
depression	sleep disorders, lethargy, excessive sadness	acupuncture, homoeopathy, music therapy, Pilates
diarrhoea	frequent evacuation of liquid faeces	breathing and relaxation, naturopathy
diverticulitis	low abdominal pain and diarrhoea or constipation	hydrotherapy, naturopathy, Western herbal medicine
eczema	itching red rash and blisters on skin	Chinese herbal medicine, naturopathy, reflexology
endometriosis	severe period and pelvic pain	acupuncture, breathing and relaxation, Chinese herbal medicine
exhaustion	extreme tiredness, lack of energy, weakness, depression	aromatherapy, meditation, music therapy
eyesight problems	e.g. short sight, long sight, eye strain, astigmatism	acupressure, Ayurveda, Bates method

fainting	loss of consciousness, light-headedness	aromatherapy, Western herbal medicine
fear	sweating, palpitations, high blood pressure	autogenic training, biofeedback training
fibrositis	pain and stiffness	acupuncture, hydrotherapy, massage, Rolfing
flatulence (wind)	excessive gas passed through mouth or anus	aromatherapy, breathing and relaxation, naturopathy
fluid retention (oedema)	accumulation of fluid in body tissues, e.g. ankles	naturopathy, Western herbal medicine
frigidity	inability to reach orgasm	dance therapy, meditation
frozen shoulder	stiff, painful shoulder joint	acupuncture, Chinese herbal medicine, chiropractic, massage
gallstones	stones in gall-bladder, possible pain, fever, vomiting	Chinese and Western herbal medicine, naturopathy
glue ear	fluid in the middle ear	cranial osteopathy, naturopathy
gout	pain and swelling in a joint, especially in toes or ears	Alexander Technique, naturopathy, t'ai chi
grief	depression, sadness, aches, headaches, fainting	art therapy, Bach flower remedies, homoeopathy
hay fever	acute nasal discharge, watery eyes, running or blocked nose	acupuncture, aromatherapy, kinesiology, naturopathy
headaches	pain in or around the head, either localized or general	aromatherapy, chiropractic, massage, reiki
heavy periods	heavy bleeding while menstruating	acupressure, acupuncture, naturopathy, Western herbal medicine
heartburn	pain in chest and perhaps acid, bitter fluid in mouth	breathing and relaxation, chiropractic, naturopathy
high blood pressure (hypertension)	dizziness, tiredness, insomnia	acupuncture, biofeedback, naturopathy, qigong

hives (nettle rash)	itching red weals on skin	homoeopathy, naturopathy, Western herbal medicine, yoga
hot flushes	flushed skin, sweating, related to menopause	acupuncture, aromatherapy, meditation, shiatsu
hyperactivity	lack of attention and lack of concentration	breathing and relaxation, cranial osteopathy
hyperventilation	breathing at very rapid rate, anxiety, hysteria	breathing and relaxation, homoeopathy, meditation
hysteria	emotional instability, tremors, paralysis	aromatherapy, breathing and relaxation, music therapy
impetigo	red patches, small pustules on face and limbs	aromatherapy, naturopathy
impotence	inability of men to have sexual intercourse	aromatherapy, autogenic training, meditation, naturopathy
insomnia	tiredness, inability to sleep	acupuncture, aromatherapy, light therapy, reiki
irritable bowel syndrome (IBS)	constipation, diarrhoea, abdominal pain	bioenergetics, massage, qigong, reflexology
laryngitis	loss of voice, cough, sometimes fever	acupuncture, aromatherapy, reflexology, Western herbal medicine
low blood pressure	dizziness, fainting, lethargy	hydrotherapy, naturopathy, Western herbal medicine
lumbago	low backache, movement may be difficult or impossible	Alexander Technique, chiropractic, osteopathy
Ménière's disease	deafness, tinnitus, vertigo, nausea and vomiting	biofeedback, homoeopathy, naturopathy
migraine	nausea, headache, flickering lights, blurring vision	Bach flower remedies, biofeedback, cranial osteopathy
morning sickness	nausea, sometimes vomiting during early pregnancy	acupressure, acupuncture, homoeopathy
mouth ulcers	break in the skin or mucous membrane of the mouth	naturopathy, Western herbal medicine

myalgic encephalomyelitis (ME)	inability to cope with anything, exhaustion, nausea	acupuncture, massage, meditation, naturopathy
nausea	feeling of wanting to vomit	acupressure, Western herbal medicine
neck pain	restricted joint movement, pain, nerve pressure	acupressure, Alexander Technique, chiropractic
neuralgia	severe burning pain in a nerve	acupuncture, healing, hydrotherapy, Western herbal medicine
night sweats (menopausal)	usually concurrent with hot flushes	aromatherapy, homoeopathy, naturopathy
obesity	high blood pressure, breathlessness, tiredness	hypnotherapy, naturopathy, Western herbal medicine
osteoarthritis	pain in the affected joint	naturopathy, osteopathy, Western herbal medicine
osteoporosis	brittle bones liable to fracture, loss of height	naturopathy, t'ai chi, Western herbal medicine, yoga
palpitations	fast beating heart, awareness of heartbeat	acupressure, biofeedback, massage, yoga
painful periods (dysmenorrhoea)	cramps in abdomen, pains before periods, headaches	acupuncture, chiropractic, naturopathy, yoga
panic attacks	acute anxiety	aromatherapy, autosuggestion, breathing and relaxation
peptic ulcer	break in lining of digestive tract, pain, bloating	acupressure, breathing and relaxation, homoeopathy
piles (haemorrhoids)	internal/external enlargement of tissue in wall of anus	acupuncture, hydrotherapy, naturopathy
post-natal depression	depression after birth, exhaustion	aromatherapy, cranial osteopathy, naturopathy, Western herbal medicine
post-traumatic stress disorder	flashbacks, sweating, nausea, palpitations	art therapy, healing, meditation, yoga
premature ejaculation	premature emission of semen	Chinese herbal medicine, hypnotherapy

LIST OF PROBLEMS AND THERAPIES FOR TREATMENT

pre-menstrual syndrome (PMS)	emotional disturbance, irritability, headaches	Chinese herbal medicine, naturopathy, reflexology
psoriasis	itchy, scaly red skin, mainly on elbows and behind knees	acupuncture, reflexology, Western herbal medicine, yoga
Raynaud's disease	white fingers, numbness, pain in fingers when they are cold	autogenic training, biofeedback, naturopathy, osteopathy
repetitive strain injury (RSI)	pain and weakness in forearm, wrist and hand	acupressure, Alexander Technique, massage
rheumatoid arthritis	inflammation of joints, pain, swelling, restricted motion	acupuncture, reflexology, t'ai chi, yoga
sciatica	pain felt down back and outer side of foot, leg or thigh	kinesiology, osteopathy, shiatsu
seasonal affective disorder (SAD)	depression, tiredness, associated with too little natural light	aromatherapy, hypnotherapy, light therapy, reflexology
shock/trauma	trembling, shallow breathing, rapid pulse, nausea, dizziness	acupuncture, art therapy, homoeopathy
sinusitis	inflammation of mucous membrane lining of sinuses	aromatherapy, homoeopathy, naturopathy, reflexology
smoking (how to give up)		aromatherapy, hypnotherapy, naturopathy, reflexology
snoring	vibration of soft palate on roof of mouth	Alexander Technique, hypnotherapy, meditation
sore throat	pain at back of mouth	hydrotherapy, naturopathy, Western herbal medicine
spots/pimples	small swelling on skin containing pus	aromatherapy, naturopathy
stammer/stutter	speech impairment	breathing and relaxation, music therapy, visualization
stress	headaches, high blood pressure, rapid pulse, aching	aromatherapy, massage, sound therapy, t'ai chi
stye	cyst on eyelid filled with pus	homoeopathy, naturopathy,
sweating (excess)	obesity, panic attacks, nervousness, fear	naturopathy, polarity therapy, Western herbal medicine

temper tantrums	anger, screaming, tears	Bach flower remedies, naturopathy
tennis elbow	inflammation of tendon of elbow	aromatherapy, chiropractic, massage, naturopathy
tension	back or neck ache, headache, depression, nausea, IBS	aromatherapy, Pilates, polarity therapy
thrush (candidiasis)	white patches on tongue, inside cheeks and in vagina	Ayurveda, hydrotherapy, naturopathy, Western herbal medicine
tinnitus	buzzing, ringing noises in ears	acupuncture, biofeedback, cranial osteopathy
vaginitis	inflammation and irritation of vagina, itching, discharge	aromatherapy, naturopathy, Western herbal medicine
varicose veins	distended veins on legs	naturopathy, Western herbal medicine, yoga
vertigo	giddiness, unsteadiness, nausea, spinning sensation	acupressure, acupuncture, Ayurveda, naturopathy
vomiting	contents of stomach ejected through the mouth	acupressure, Western herbal medicine
warts	growth on skin surface on hands, face, feet and genitals	aromatherapy, homoeopathy, hypnotherapy
whiplash	sprained ligaments in neck	chiropractic, healing, osteopathy

Part IV
USEFUL INFORMATION

NATIONAL ORGANIZATIONS

The following pages comprise a detailed list of organizations in alphabetical order under the following countries: Australia, Canada, Ireland, New Zealand, South Africa, United Kingdom, United States of America.

Each organization is listed with address, phone number, fax and email, in that order. Every effort has been made to ensure that each organization listed is reputable and to obtain as many details as possible.

'General' organizations are national organizations that relate to all or a number of alternative therapies. These are followed by organizations for each therapy described in this book. Sometimes they are national and sometimes local to a large area. If there is no organization listed for the therapy you require, contact one of the general organizations.

General

Australia

Australasian College of Advancement in Medicine
P O Box 5119
Erina Fair
NSW 2250
043 249 302
043 249 350
acam@enternet.com.au

Australasian College of Natural Therapies
57 Foveaux Street
Surrey Hills
NSW 2010
029 211 7744
029 281 4411
info@acnt.edu.au

Australian College of Mind/Body Medicine
81 Ormond Road
Elwood 3184
016 378 483
039 525 6639

Australian Complementary Health Association
247 Flinders Lane
Melbourne 3000
039 650 5327
039 650 8404

Australian Institute of Holistic Medicine
P O Box 3079
Jandkot
WA 6164
019 417 3553
019 417 1881

Australian Natural Therapists Association
P O Box 856
Caloundra
QLD 4551
075 491 9850

Australian Traditional Medicine Society
Suite 3
First Floor
120 Blaxland Road
Ryde
NSW 2122
029 809 6800
029 809 7570

Canada

Canadian Holistic Healing Association
1644 W Broadway
Suite 210
Vancouver
VA V6J 1X6
604 736 6727

Canadian Holistic Medical Association
42 Redpath Avenue
Toronto
ON M4S 2J6
416 485 3071

New Zealand

Canterbury College of Natural Medicine
P O Box 4529
Christchurch
03 366 0373
03 366 5342

New Zealand Register of Complementary Health Practitioners
c/o New Zealand Health Network
P O Box 337
Christchurch
02 531 0709

Wellpark College of Natural Therapies
P O Box 78–229
Grey Lynn
Auckland
09 360 0560
09 376 4307

South Africa

Complementary Health Initiative
P O Box 1195
North Riding 2162
Johannesburg
011 462 6233
011 462 6233

Confederation of Complementary Health Associations of South Africa
P O Box 2471
Clareinch 7740
021 588 709

South African Complementary Medical Association
P O Box 18558
Wynberg 7824
021 797 8912
021 797 6026

UK

Association of Holistic Practitioners International
Flat 8
Soar Court Scott Street
Tenewydd
Rhondda CF42 5NA
01443 771804

British Complementary Medicine Association
249 Fosse Road South
Leicester LE3 1AE
0116 282 5511

British Register of Complementary Medicine
P O Box 194
London SE16 1QZ
0171 237 6175
0171 237 6175

Complementary Medical Association
The Meridian
142a Greenwich High Road
London SE10 8NN
studio@hawk-in.demon.co.uk

Council for Complementary and Alternative Medicine
Park House
206–208 Latimer Road
London W10 6RE
0181 968 3862

Federation of Holistic Therapists
38a Portsmouth Road
Woolston
Southampton SO19 9AD
01703 422695

Guild of Complementary Practitioners
Liddell House
Liddell Close
Finchampstead
Berkshire RG40 4NS
0118 973 5757
0118 973 5767

Institute for Complementary Medicine (ICM)
Unit 15
Tavern Quay
Commercial Centre
Rope Street
London SE16 1TX
0171 237 5165
0171 237 5175

Research Council for Complementary Medicine
60 Great Ormond Street
London WC1N 3JF
0171 833 8897
0171 278 7412
rccm@gn.apc.org

USA

American Academy of Environmental Medicine
Box CN 1001–2001
New Hope
PA 18938
215 862 4544
215 862 4583
aaem@bellatlantic.net

American College for Advancement in Medicine
23121 Verdugo Drive
Suite 204
Laguna Hills
CA 92653
acam@acam.org

American Holistic Medical Association
6728 Old McLean Village Drive
McLean
VA 223101-3906
703 556 9728
703 556 8729
HolistMed@aol.com

American Holistic Nurses' Association
P O Box 2130
Flagstaff
AZ 86003-2130

Foundation for Alternative Medicine
160 NW Widmer Place
Albany
OR 97321
503 926 4678

Foundation for East–West Medicine
2512 Manoa Road
Honolulu
HI 96822
808 946 2069
808 946 0378

Holistic Health Association
P O Box 17400
Anaheim
CA 92817–7400
714 779 6152

Institute for Holistic Education
33719 116th Street Box SH
Twin Lakes
WI 53181
414 889 8501

National Association of Certified Natural Health Professionals
810 S Buffalo Street
Warsaw
IN 46580
800 321 1005
219 269 4060

Natural Alternative Center Inc
310 West 72nd Street
New York
NY 10023
212 580 3333

New Mexico College of Natural Healing
P O Box 211
3030 Pinos Altos Road
Silver City
NM 88062
505 538 0050
nmenh@plata.com

People's Medical Society
462 Walnut Street
Allentown
PA 18102
800 624 8773

Acupressure

Canada

British Columbia Acupressure Therapists' Association
718 Wallace Crescent
Comox
BC V9M 3V8
bcata@islandnet.com

Canadian Acupressure Institute Inc
301–733 Johnson Street
Victoria
BC V8W 3C7
250 388 7475
250 383 3647
caii@tnet.net

USA

Acupressure Institute
1533 Shattuck Avenue
Berkeley
CA 94709
510 845 1059
info@acupressure.com

American Oriental Bodywork Association
6801 Jericho Turnpike
Syosset
NY 11791
516 364 5533

Jin Shino Do Foundation for Bodymind Acupressure
1084G San Miguel Canyon Road
Watsonville
CA 95076
408 763 7702
408 763 1551

Acupuncture

Australia

Australian Acupuncture Association Ltd
P O Box 5142, West End
Brisbane
QLD 4101
073 846 5866
073 846 5276
aaca@eis.net.au

Australian College of Acupuncturists
5 Georgette Crescent
Endeavour Hills
VIC 3802
039 480 2130

Canada

Acupuncture Foundation of Canada Institute
2131 Lawrence Avenue E
Suite 204
Scarborough
ON M1R 5G4
416 752 3988
416 752 4398
info@afcinstitute.com

Canadian Medical Acupuncture Society
9904–106 Street NW
Edmonton
AB T5K 1C4
403 426 2760
403 426 5650

South Africa

Acupuncture Association
3 Tana Road
Emmarentia
011 888 3071
082 457 2259

Acupuncture Association of the Western Cape
P O Box 39
Edgemead 7441
021 949 3232

South African Medical Acupuncture Society
021 885 1010
021 885 1565

Western Cape Su Jok Acupuncture Institute
3 Periwinkle Close
Kommetjie 7975
021 783 34460

UK

Association of Chinese Acupuncture
Prospect House
2 Grove Lane
Retford
Nottinghamshire
DN22 6NA
01777 704411
01777 704411

British Acupuncture Council
Park House
206–208 Latimer Road
London W10 6RE
0181 964 0222
0181 964 0333

British Medical Acupuncture Society
Newton House, Newton Lane
Whitley, Warrington
Cheshire WA4 4JA
01925 730727
01925 730492
Bmasadmin@aol.com

USA

American Academy of Medical Acupuncture
5820 Wilshire Boulevard
Suite 500
Los Angeles
CA 90036
323 937 5514

American Association of Acupuncture and Bio-Energetic Medicine
2512 Manoa Road
Honolulu
HI 96822
808 946 2069
808 946 0378

American College of Acupuncture & Oriental Medicine
9100 Park West Drive
Houston
TX 77063
713 780 9777
713 781 5781
webmaster@acaom.edu

California Association of Acupuncture and Oriental Medicine
1231 State Street
Suite 208A
Santa Barbara
CA 93101
805 957 4384
805 957 4389

Council of Colleges of Acupuncture & Oriental Medicine
8403 Colesville Road
Suite 370
Silver Spring
MD 20910
301 608 9175
301 608 9576

Minnesota Institute of Acupuncture & Herbal Studies
1821 University Avenue
W Suite 278-S
St Paul
MN 55104
651 603 0994
miahs@millcomm.com

National Association of Teachers of Acupuncture and Oriental Medicine
2525 South Madison
Denver
CO 80210
303 329 6355

National Acupuncture Foundation
1718 M Street
Suite 195
Washington
DC 20036
202 332 5794

National Acupuncture and Oriental Medicine Alliance
14637 Starr Road SE
Olalla
WA 98359
206 851 6896
206 851 6883

National Commission for the Certification of Acupuncturists
1424 16th Street NW
Washington
DC 20036
202 232 1404

Alexander Technique

Australia

Alexander Technique International
11/11 Stanley Street
Darlinghurst
NSW 2010
029 331 7563
australia@ati-net.com

Australian Society of Teachers of the Alexander Technique
P O Box 716
Darlinghurst
Sydney
NSW 2010
039 510 5788
greg@sydney.dialix.oz.au

Canada

Canadian Society of Teachers of the Alexander Technique
P O Box 47025
19–555 West 12th Avenue
Vancouver
BC V5Z 3XO

Ireland

Alexander Technique International
13 Bru Na Mara
Fort Lorenzo
Galway
091 526326

South Africa

South African Society of Teachers of the Alexander Technique
5 Leinster Road
Green Point 8001
Cape Town

UK

Alexander Technique International
66C Thurlestone Road
West Norwood,
London SE27 0PD
uk@ati-net.com

Society of Teachers of the Alexander Technique
20 London House
266 Fulham Road
London SW10 9EL
0171 351 0828
0171 352 1556

USA

Alexander Foundation
605 West Phil-Ellena Street
Philadelphia
PA 19119
215 844 0670
215 844 0670

Alexander Technique International
1692 Massachusetts Avenue
Third Floor
Cambridge
MA 02138
617 497 2242
617 497 2615
usa@ati-net.com

American Center for the Alexander Technique
129 West 67th Street
New York
NY 10023–9998
212 799 0468

North American Society of Teachers of the Alexander Technique
3010 Hennepin Avenue South
Suite 10
Minneapolis
MIN 55408
612 824 5066
612 822 7224
nastat@ix.netcom.com

Anthroposophical medicine

South Africa

Anthroposophical Medicine Association of South Africa
021 762 2364
021 761 1973

UK

Anthroposophical Medical Association
Park Attwood Therapeutic Centre
Trimpley
Bewdley
Worcestershire DY12 1RE
01299 861444

Anthroposophical Society of Great Britain
Rudolph Steiner House
35 Park Road
London NW1 6XT
0171 723 4400
0171 724 4364

Association of Eurythmy Therapists
Rudolf Steiner House
35 Park Road
London NW1 6XT
0171 723 4400
0171 724 4364

USA

Physician's Association for Anthroposophical Medicine
7953 California Avenue
Fair Oaks
CA 95628
916 967 8250
916 966 5314

Aromatherapy

Australia

International Federation of Aromatherapists
1/390 Burwood Road
Hawthorn
VIC 3122
039 530 0067

Canada

British Columbia Association of Practicing Aromatherapists
11–1328 West 73rd Avenue
Vancouver
BC V6P 3E7
604 267 9745
604 267 9746

Canadian Federation of Aromatherapists
The Village Arcade
50 Cumberland Street
Box 18
Toronto
ON M4W 1J5
416 961 9445
416 961 5547

Canadian National School of Aromatherapy
2604 Hornsgate Drive
Mississauga
ON L5K 1P6
905 823 9581
905 823 7265
cnsa@ica.net

South Africa

Association of Aromatherapists
P O Box 23924
Claremont 7735
021 531 7314
021 531 7314

UK

Aromatherapy Trade Council
P O Box 52
Leicester LE16 8ZX
01858 465731
01858 465731

Aromatherapy Organizations Council
3 Latymer Close
Braybrooke
Market Harborough
Leicester LE16 8LN
01858 434242

International Federation of Aromatherapists
Stamford House
2–4 Chiswick High Road
London W4 1TH
0181 742 2605

International Society of Professional Aromatherapists
ISPA House
82 Ashby Road
Hinkley
Leicestershire LE10 1SN
01455 637987

School of Holistic Aromatherapy
108B Haverstock Hill
London NW3 2BD
0171 284 1315

Shirley Price Aromatherapy Ltd
Essentia House
Upper Bond Street
Hinckley
Leicestershire LE10 1RS
01455 615466

Tisserand Institute
65 Church Road
Hove
East Sussex BN3 2BD
01273 206640

USA

American Alliance of Aromatherapy
P O Box 309
Depoe Bay
OR 97341
800 809 9850
800 809 9808

Atlantic Institute of Aromatherapy
16018 Saddlestring Drive
Tampa
FL 33618

USEFUL INFORMATION

National Association of Holistic Aromatherapy
P O Box 17622
Boulder
CO 80308-0622
303 258 3791

Art therapy

Canada

Canadian Art Therapy Association – Eastern Chapter
2400 Dundas Street W
Unit 6
Suite 601
Mississauga
ON L5K 2R8
905 469 9442

Canadian Art Therapy Association – Western Chapter
350–1425 Marine Drive
West Vancouver
BC V7T 1B9
604 926 9381

Le Association des Art-Therapeutes du Quebec
5764 avenue Monkland
bureau 301
Montreal
QU H4A 1E9
514 990 5415
514 483 6692

UK

Art Therapy
Centre for Psychotherapeutic Studies
14 Claremont Crescent
Sheffield S10 2TA
0114 222 2967

British Association of Art Therapists
11a Richmond Road
Brighton BN2 3RL
0171 383 3774
0171 387 5513

USA

American Art Therapy Association
1202 Allanson Road
Mundelein
IL 60060
847 949 6064
847 566 4580
estygariii@aol.com

National Coalition of Arts Therapies Associations
2000 Century Plaza
Suite 108
Columbia
MD 21044
410 997 4040
410 997 4048

Autogenic training

UK
British Association for Autogenic Training and Therapy
c/o Royal London Homoeopathic Hospital NHS Trust
Great Ormond Street
London WC1N 3HR
0171 837 8833
0171 833 7269

Centre for Autogenic Training (South West)
The Old Dairy
2 Coombe Lane
Torquay
Devon TQ2 8DY
01803 312098

USA
Mind Body Health Sciences
393 Dixon Road
Boulder
CO 80302

Auto-suggestion

Contact a national Hypnotherapy organization for further information (see p. 180).

Ayurveda

Australia
Maharishi Ayurveda Health Centre
P O Box 81
Bundoora
VIC 3083

South Africa
South African Ayurvedic Medical Association
012 448 9366
012 348 9365

South African Ayurvedic Medicine Association
85 Harvey Road
Morningside
Durban 4001
031 303 3245
021 871 1777

UK
The Association of Accredited Ayurvedic Practitioners
50 Penywern Road
London SW5 9SX
0171 370 2255
0171 370 5157

USA
American Institute of Vedic Studies
PO Box 8357
Santa Fe
NM 87504–8357
505 983 9385
505 982 5807

Ayurveda at Spirit Rest
P O Box 3537
Pagosa Springs
CO 81147–3537
970 264 2573

Ayurveda Holistic Center
82 Bayville Ave
Bayville
NY 11709
516 628 8200
516 628 8200
ayurvedahc@holistic.com

Ayurvedic Institute
11311 Menaul NE
Suite A
Albuquerque
NM 87112
505 291 9698

Ayurvedic Medicine of New York
13 West Ninth Street
New York
NY 10011
212 505 8971
212 677 5397
drgerson@att.net

John Douillard's Ayurvedic LifeSpa
3065 Center Green Drive
Suite 110
Boulder
CO 80301
303 442 1164
303 442 1240
LifeSpa@aol.com

Lotus Ayurvedic Center
4145 Clares Street
Suite D
Capitola
CA 95010
408 479 1667

National Institute of Ayurvedic Medicine
584 Milltown Road
Brewster
NY 10509
914 278 8700 (fax)

Vinayak Ayurveda Center
2509 Virginia NE
Suite D
Albuquerque
NM 87110
505 296 6522
505 298 2932

Bates method for better eyesight

Australia

Australian Optometrical Association
26 Ridge Road
North Sydney
029 922 2566

UK

Bates Association of Great Britain
P O Box 25
Shoreham by Sea
Sussex BN43 6ZF
01273 422090
01273 279983

USA

American Optometry Association
Communications Center
243 North Lindbergh Boulevard
St Louis
MO 63141
314 991 4100
314 991 4101

Cambridge Institution for Better Vision
65 Wenham Road
Topsfield
MA 01983
508 887 3883

College of Optometrists in Vision Development
P O Box 285
Chula Vista
CA 91912–0285
619 425 6191

Natural Vision International Ltd
P O Box 157
Manitowoc
WI 54221
800 255 4715

Bioenergetics

Canada

Atlantic Canada Society for Bioenergetic Analysis
Chrysalis Bioenergetic Centre
Box 1147
143 Mount Edward Road
Charlottetown
PE C1A 7N5
902 894 3244
bdoyle@isn.net

UK

Scottish Centre for Bioenergetic Analysis
c/o David Campbell
Davison Clinic/Charing Cross Mansions
12 St George's Road
Glasgow G3 6UJ
0141 332 6371

USA

International Institute for Bioenergetic Analysis
144 East 36th Street
Apartment 1A
New York
NY 10016
212 532 7742

Biofeedback training

UK

Aleph One Ltd
The Old Courthouse
Bottisham
Cambridge CB5 9BA
01223 811679
01223 812713
info@aleph1.co.uk

Biomonitors
2 Old Garden Court
Mount Pleasant
St Albans
Hertfordshire AL3 4QR
01727 833882

USA

Association for Applied Psychophysiology and Biofeedback
10200 West 44th Avenue
Suite 304
Wheat Ridge
CO 80033–2840
303 422 8436
303 422 8894
AAPB@resourcenter.com

Biofeedback Society of California
P O Box 4384
Huntington Beach
CA 92605–4384
714 848 0022
ba588@lafn.org

Bio Research Institute
331 East Cotati Avenue
Cotati
CA 94931
707 795 2460
707 795 2460
bri@7hz.com

Pennsylvania Society for Behavioral Medicine & Biofeedback
1616 Walnut Street
Suite 2114
Philadelphia
PA 19103
215 545 7708

Buteyko method

USA

Respiratory Health Institute
90 Park Avenue, Suite 1700
New York
NY 10016
212 984 0762
212 984 1861
smerkin@interserv.com

Chiropractic

Australia

Chiropractors' Association of Australia
459 Great Western Highway
Faulconbridge
NSW 2776
061 247 515644
061 247 515856
caa_nat@pnc.com.au

Canada

Canadian Chiropractic Association
1396 Eglinton Avenue W
Toronto
ON M6R 2H2
416 781 5656
416 781 7344
ccachiro@inforamp.net

World Federation of Chiropractic
78 Glencairn Avenue
Toronto
ON M4R 1M8
416 484 9978
416 484 9665
worldfed@sympatico.ca

Ireland

Chiropractic Association of Ireland
28 Fair Street
Drogheda
County Louth
041 305999
041 51863

New Zealand

Mt Maunganui Chiropractic Centre Ltd
41 Golf Road
Mt Maunganui 3002
647 575 9567
647 575 9567
mark@chiropractic.co.nz

New Zealand Chiropractors' Association
P O Box 7144
Wellesley Street
Auckland
064 9373 4343
064 9373 5973

South Africa

Chiropractors, Homeopaths and Allied Health Professions Council of South Africa
012 324 4640
012 324 4642

UK

British Association for Applied Chiropractic
The Old Post Office
Cherry Street
Stratton Audley
Nr Bicester
Oxfordshire OX6 9BA
01869 277111
01869 277111

British Chiropractic Association
Blagrave House
17 Blagrave Street
Reading RG1 1QB
01189 505950
01189 588946

McTimoney Chiropractic Association
21 High Street
Eynsham
Oxon OX8 1HE
01865 880974
01865 880975

Scottish Chiropractic Association
St Boswell's Clinic
Main Street
St Boswell's
Scotland TD6 0AP

USA

American Chiropractic Association
1701 Claredon Boulevard
Arlington
VA 22209
703 276 8800
703 243 2593

USEFUL INFORMATION

American Veterinary Chiropractic Association
Animal Chiropractic Center
623 Main
Hillsdale
IL 61257
309 658 2920
309 658 2622

World Chiropractic Alliance
2950 North Dobson Road
Suite 1
Chandler
AR 85224–1802
602 732 9313 (fax)

Colour therapy

UK

Hygeia Studios
Brook House
Avening, Tetbury
Gloucestershire GL8 8NS
01453 832150
01453 832150

Crystal and Gem therapies

UK

Affiliation of Crystal Healing Organizations
P O Box 344
Manchester M60 2EZ
0161 278 0096

International Association of Crystal Healing Therapists
Unit 19
The Corn Exchange
Manchester

USA

Gemology Stuff
PO Box 1132
Pismo Beach
CA 93448
805 773 0101
805 773 4288

Dance therapy

UK

Association for Dance Movement Therapy
c/o Arts Therapies Department
Springfield Hospital
Glenburnie Road
Tooting
London SW17 7DJ
0181 672 9911

Creative Therapy Unit
The Briars
Crabb Lane
Exeter EX2 9JD
01392 221241

Medau Society
8b Robson House
East Street
Epsom
Surrey KT17 1HH
01372 729056

USA

American Dance Therapy
Association
2000 Century Plaza
Suite 108
10632 Little Patuxent Parkway
Columbia
MD 21044-3265
410 997 4040
410 997 4048
info@adta.org

Feldenkrais method

UK

Feldenkrais Centre
P O Box 370
London N10 3XA
0181 346 0258

USA

Feldenkrais Guild of North America
524 Ellsworth Street SW
P O Box 489
Albany
OR 97321-0143
541 926 0981
541 926 0572
Webmaster@FGNA

Flotation therapy

Australia

Keturah Bodycare
5–7/500 Beaufort Street
Highgate
Perth
WA 6003
089 228 0855
089 228 0850
kit@keturah.com.au

South Africa

Still Point Relaxation Centre
36 Collingwood Road
Observatory 7925
021 448 3353
021 448 3360
stillpnt@gem.co.za

UK

Flotation Tank Association
PO Box 11024
London SW4 7ZF
0171 627 4962

USA

Stresslab
Flotation and Massage Therapy
  Services
7 Chester Avenue
Medford
NJ 08055
609 654 0442

Flower remedies

Canada
Canadian Wild Flower Society
75 Ternhill Crescent
Don Mills
ONT M3C

New Zealand
Bach Flower Remedies
Box 358 Waiuku
09 235 7057
bachnz@ps.gen.nz

UK
Dr Edward Bach Foundation
Mount Vernon
Sotwell
Wallingford
Oxfordshire OX10 0PZ
01491 834678

Flower Essence Fellowship
Laurel Farm Clinic
17 Carlingscott
Peasdown St John
Bath
01761 434098

USA
Dr Edward Bach Healing Society
644 Marrick Road
Lynbrook
NY 11563
516 593 2206

Healing

Australia
Australian Spiritual Healers Association
P O Box 4073
Eight Mile Plains
Queensland 4113

Canada
National Federation of Spiritual Healers (Canada)
TH 64/331
Military Trail
West Hill
Scarborough
ON M1E 4E3

New Zealand
New Zealand Federation of Spiritual Healers Inc
P O Box 9502
Newmarket
Auckland 1

UK
British Alliance of Healing Associations
3 Sandy Lane
Gisleham
Lowestoft
Suffolk NR33 8EQ
01502 742224

British Alliance of Healing Organizations
23 Nutcroft Grove
Fetcham
Leatherhead
Surrey KT22 9LA
01372 373241

Confederation of Healing Organizations
The Red and White House
113 High Street
Berkhamstead
Herts HP4 2DJ
01442 870660

National Federation of Spiritual Healers
Old Manor Farm Studio
Church Street
Sunbury on Thames
Middlesex TW16 6RG
01932 783164
01932 779648
office@nfsh.org.uk

USA

Association for Research and Enlightenment
P O Box 595
Virginia Beach
VA 23451

Healing Buddha Foundation
P O Box 87
Sebastopol
CA 95472
707 823 8700
707 823 8787
buddhaheal@aol.com

Hellerwork

USA

Hellerwork International
406 Berry Street
Mount Shasta
CA 96067
916 926 3500
916 926 6839
hellerwork@hellerwork.com

Herbal medicine – Chinese

UK

Register of Chinese Herbal Medicine
PO Box 400
Wembley
Middlesex HA9 9NZ
0171 224 0803

USA

Rocky Mountain Herbal Institute
P O Box 579
Hot Springs
MN 59845
406 741 3811
rmhi@rmhiherbal.org

# Herbal medicine – Western

Australia

Australian Herb Society Inc
P O Box 110
Mapleton
Queensland 4560
075 446 9243
075 446 9277

National Herbalists Association of Australia
P O Box 61
Broadway
NSW 2007
029 211 6437
029 211 6452
nhaa@org.au

Canada

Canadian Association of Herbal Practitioners
921 17th Avenue SW
Calgary
AB T2T 0A4

Ontario Herbalists' Association
11 Winthrop Place
Stoney Creek
ON L8G 3M7
416 536 1509
416 536 1509

New Zealand

Aotearoa Herbalists Inc
Horahora Road
RD1
Putaruru

Herb Federation of New Zealand
P O Box 4055
Nelson South
03 546 9121
03 546 9121

UK

National Institute of Medical Herbalists
56 Longbrook Street
Exeter EX4 6AH
01392 426022
01392 498963

College of Phytotherapy
Bucksteep Manor
Bodle Street Green
Hailsham
East Sussex BN27 4RJ
01323 834800

USA

American Herbalists Guild
PO Box 70
Roosevelt
UT 84066
435 722 8434
435 722 8452
ahgoffice@earthlink.net

Herb Research Foundation
1007 Pearl Street
Suite 200
Boulder
CO 80302
303 449 7849
303 449 2265
herbal@netcom.com

Minnesota Institute of Acupuncture & Herbal Studies
1821 University Avenue
W Suite 278-S
St Paul
MN 55104
651 603 0994
miahs@millcomm.com

Homoeopathy

Australia

Australian Homoeopathic Association
7 Munro Street
Auchenflower
Queensland 4066
029 879 0049
georgec@uq.edu.au

Victorian Register of Certified Homoeopathic Practitioners
3 Willow Street
Preston
VIC 3072
039 484 6048
039 521 3596

Canada

National United Professional Association of Trained Homeopaths (Canada)
1960 Boake Street
Orleans
ON K4A 3K1
613 834 2516
613 834 2517
rudi@web.net

Ontario Homeopathic Association
P O Box 258
Station P
Toronto
ON M5S 2Z2
416 488 9685
416 481 4444
oha@istar.ca

SPHQ (Syndicat Professionnel des Homeopathes du Quebec)
1600 De Lorimier
Local 295
Montreal
QC H2K 3W5
514 525 2037
514 525 1299

Vancouver Centre for Homeopathy
2246 Spruce Street
Vancouver
BC V6H 2P3

Calgary Centre for Homeopathy
1040–14th Avenue SW
Calgary
AL T2R 0P1
403 245 8558

New Zealand

New Zealand Institute of Classical Homoeopathy
24 Westhaven Drive
Tawa
Wellington

NZ Homoeopathic Society Inc
P O Box 67–095
Mount Eden
Auckland

USEFUL INFORMATION

South Africa

Chiropractors, Homeopaths and Allied Health Service
Professions Council of South Africa
012 324 4640
012 324 4640

Homeopathic Association
011 393 3427
012 348 9366

South African Homeopathic Medical Association
012 348 9366
012 348 9365

UK

Faculty of Homoeopathy
2 Powis Place
London WC1N 3HT
0171 566 7800

Register of Homoeopathic Practitioners
32 King Edward Road
Swansea SA1 4LL
01792 655886

Society of Homoeopaths
2 Artizan Road
Northampton NN1 4HU
01604 621400
01604 622622
society of homoeopaths@btinternet.com

United Kingdom Homoeopathic Medical Association
6 Livingstone Road
Gravesend
Kent DA12 5DZ
01474 560336

USA

Homeopathic Academy of Naturopathic Physicians
12132 SE Foster Place
Portland
OR 97266
503 761 3298
503 762 1929
hanp@igc.apc.org

International Foundation for Homeopathy
P O Box 7
Edmonds
WA 98020
425 776 4147
425 776 1499
ifh@nwlink.com

National Center for Homeopathy
801 North Fairfax Street
Suite 306
Alexandria
VA 22314
703 548 7790
703 548 7792
nchinfo@igc.apc.org

Hydrotherapy

Switzerland

International School of Colon Hydrotherapy
IMI-Lientalerhof
3723 Kiental-CH
011 41 33 676 2676

UK

Colonic International Association
16 Drumond Drive
Tring
Hertfordshire HP23 5DE
01442 827687

UK College of Hydrotherapy
515 Hagley Road
Birmingham B66 4AX
0121 429 9191

USA

International Association for Colon Hydrotherapy
P O Box 461285
San Antonio
TX 78246–1285
210 366 2888
210 366 2999
iact@healthy.net

International Spa & Fitness Association (ISPA)
1300 L Street NW
Suite 1050
Washington DC 20005–4107
202 789 5920
202 898 0484

Hypnotherapy

Australia

Australian Academy of Hypnotic Science
Kordover House
114–116 Church Street
Hawthorn
VIC 3122
039 888 6203
039 9815 0047
admin@aahs.com.au

Australian Society of Clinical Hypnotherapists
38 Denistone Road
P O Box 471
Eastwood
NSW 2122
029 874 2776
029 554 4742
briggs@flex.com.au

Australian Society of Hypnosis
Austin Hospital
Heidelberg
VIC 3084

Canada

Canadian Society of Hypnosis
Labelle
7027 Edgemont Drive
Calgary
Alberta T3A 2H9

UK

Association of Ethical and Professional Hypnotherapists
181 The Downs
Harlow
Essex CM20 3RH
01279 425284
01279 320479
rscollege@aol.com

British Society of Medical and Dental Hypnosis
17 Keppel View Road
Kimberworth
Rotherham
South Yorkshire S61 2AR
01709 554558

National Register of Hypnotherapists and Psychotherapists
12 Cross Street
Nelson
Lancashire BB9 7EN
01282 699378
01282 698633

National School of Hypnosis and Psychotherapy
28 Finsbury Park Road
London N4 2JX
0171 359 6991

USA

American Institute of Hypnotherapy
16842 Von Karman
Apartment 475
Irvine
CA 91724
714 261 6400
aih@hypnosis.com

International Medical and Dental Hypnotherapy Association
4110 Edgeland
Suite 800
Royal Oak
MI 48073–2285
248 549 5594
800 257 5467

Iridology

Australia

Herbal Happiness
15 Fitzmaurice Street
Kaleen, Canberra
ACT 2617
026 241 5193
026 241 0980
vicoates@pcug.com.au

Canada

Canadian Neuro-Optic Research Institute
2078 Wascana Street
Regina
Saskatchewan S4T 4J7
306 359 7694
306 525 2659

Iridologist Association of Canada
5150 Dundas Street W
Suite 201
Etobicoke
ON M9A 1C3

UK

Guild of Naturopathic Iridologists
94 Grosvenor Road
London SW1V 3LF
0171 834 3579

International Association of Clinical Iridologists
Orchard Villa
Porters Park Drive
Shenley
Hertfordshire WD7 9DS
01923 856222
01923 857670

Society of Iridologists
998 Wimbourne Road
Bournemouth BH9 2DE
01202 518078

Kinesiology

Australia

Australian Kinesiology Association
P O Box 155
Ormond 3204
039 578 9322
039 578 1468

International Association of Specialised Kinesiologists
P O Box 850
Ringwood 3134
039 879 3357

UK

Academy & Association of Systematic Kinesiology
39 Browns Road
Surbiton
Surrey KT5 8ST
0181 399 3215
0181 390 1010

International College of Applied Kinesiology
Downsview
New Hall Lane
Small Dole
West Sussex BN5 9YJ

Kinesiology Foundation
P O Box 7891
London SW19 1ZB
0181 545 1255

USA

International College of Applied Kinesiology
PO Box 905
Lawrence
KS 66044–0905
913 542 1801

Light therapy

UK

Light and Sound Therapy Centre
90 Queen Elizabeth's Walk
London N16 5UQ
0181 880 1269

Seasonal Affective Disorder Association (SADA)
P O Box 989
Steyning BN44 3HG
01903 814942

USA

College of Syntonic Optometry
1200 Robeson Street
Fall River
MA 02720–5508
508 673 1251

National Organization for Seasonal Affective Disorder (NOSAD)
P O Box 40190
Washington DC 20016

Society for Light Treatment and Biological Rhythms (SLTBR)
10200 West 44th Avenue
Suite 304
Wheat Ridge
CO 80033–2840
303 424 3697
303 422 8894
sltbr@resourcenter.com

Massage

Australia

Massage Association of Australia
P O Box 1187
Camberwell
VIC 3124
039 885 7631
039 886 9095
info@maa.org.au

Association of Massage Therapists
18a Spit Road
Mosman
NSW 1088
039 510 3930

Convocation of Massage Therapists – Australia
55 Springfield Avenue
Kotara
NSW 2289
024 957 4095
024 957 2232

Massage Australia
P O Box 38
Wentworth Falls
NSW 2782
024 757 3050
024 757 3936

Canada

Association of Physiotherapists and Massage Practitioners of BC
Suite 103
1089 West Broadway
Vancouver
BC V6H 0V3

Canadian Massage Therapist Alliance
365 Bloor Street E
Suite 1807
Toronto
ON M4W 3L4
416 968 2149
416 968 6818
cmta@collinscan.com

South Africa

Holistic Massage Practitioners Association
021 782 5909

UK

British Massage Therapy Council
2 Layer Gardens
London W3 9PR
0181 992 2554

London College of Massage
5 Newman Passage
London W1P 3PF
0171 323 3574
0171 637 7125

Scottish Massage Therapists Organization
70 Lochside Road
Denmore Park
Bridge of Don
Aberdeen AB23 8QW
01224 822956

USA

American Massage Therapy Association
820 Davis Street
Suite 100
Evanston
IL 60201-4444
847 864 0123
847 864 1178

American Institute of Massage Therapy Inc
2101 N Federal Highway
Fort Lauderdale
FL 33334
800 752 2793

Association of Bodywork and Massage Professionals
28677 Buffalo Park Road
Evergreen
CO 80439-7347
303 674 8478
303 674 0859

International Association of Infant Massage
P O Box 438
Elma
New York 14059-0438
716 652 9789
716 652 1990

International Massage Association
3000 Connecticut Avenue NW
Suite 102
Washington
DC 20008
202 387 6555
202 332 0531

USEFUL INFORMATION **185**

Medical astrology

UK

Centre for Psychological Astrology
P O Box 890
London NW5 2NE

Company of Astrologers
6 Queen Square
London WC1
0171 837 5510

USA

Astro-Analytics
16440 Haynes Street
Van Nuys
CA 91406

Astrosonics
Route 4
P O Box 288
Los Lunas
NM 87031

Meditation

Australia

Australian Buddhist Network
Buddhist Federation of Australia
PO Box K1020
Haymarket
NSW 2010
029 9212 3071
bfa@pobox.com

National Office World Plan Executive Council of Australia
Maharishi Vedic College
039 467 3235
robbrown@eisa.net.au

New Zealand

Auckland Buddhist Centre
PO 78–205
Grey Lynn
Auckland
09 378 1120

Auckland Buddhist Vihara
29 Harris Road
Mt Wellington
Auckland
09 579 443

Maharishi Foundation of New Zealand
09 426 4567
09 426 4563

Wellington Buddhist Centre
PO Box 12–311
Wellington North
Wellington
04 386 3940

UK

School of Meditation
158 Holland Park Avenue
London W11 4UH
0171 603 6116

Transcendental Meditation
Freepost
London SW1 4YY
0800 269303

Transcendental Meditation
4 West Newington Place
Edinburgh EH9 1QT
0131 668 1649
0131 662 4992

USA

Dharma Net International
PO Box 4951
Berkeley
CA 94704-4951
dharma@dharmanet.org

**Maharishi Vedic School and
  Maharishi Ayur-Veda School**
234 South 22nd Street
Philadelphia
PA 19103
215 732 8464
kkliens@erols.com

TM Program for Delaware County
328 Prospect Avenue
Clifton Heights
PA 19018
610 622 9977
tmdelco@erols.com

**Transcendental Meditation
Group Program Facility**
2320 South Eads Street
Arlington
VA 22202
703 486 2222 (fax)

Metamorphic technique

UK

UK Metamorphic Association
67 Ritherdon Road
Tooting
London SW17 8QE
0181 672 5951
0181 672 5951

USA

The Metamorphic Technique
Sebastopol
CA
707 824 0527
707 522 8674

Music therapy

Australia

**Australian Music Therapy
  Association (AMTA)**
8 Williamson Road
Box Hill
North Victoria 3129
039 898 5570
039 345 5090
shoemarh@cryptic.rch.unimelb.edu.au

Canada

**Canadian Association for Music
  Therapy/Association de
  Musicotherpaie du Canada**
Wilfrid Laurier University
Waterloo
ON N2L 3C5
519 884 1970 ext 6828
519 884 8853
ltracy@machl.wlu.ca

UK

**Association of Professional
  Music Therapists**
Chestnut Cottage, 38 Pierce Lane
Fulbourn
Cambridge CB1 5DL
01223 880377

USEFUL INFORMATION

British Society for Music Therapy (BSMT)
25 Rosslyn Avenue
East Barnet
Hertfordshire EN4 8DH
0181 368 8879
0181 368 8879

Nordoff-Robbins Music Therapy Centre
2 Lissenden Gardens
London NW5 1PP
0171 267 4496

USA

American Association for Music Therapy
1 Station Plaza
Ossining, NY 10562
914 944 9260
914 944 9387

American Music Therapy Assocation Inc
8455 Colesville Road
Suite 1000
Silver Springs
MD 20910
301 589 3300
301 589 5175
info@musictherapy.org

National Association of Music Therapy
8455 Colesville Road
Suite 930
Silver Springs
MD 20910
301 589 3300

Naturopathy

Australia

Australian Naturopathic Practitioners Association
First Floor
609–611 Camberwell Road
Camberwell
VIC 3124
039 889 0334
039 889 0334

Canada

Canadian College of Naturopathic Medicine
2300 Yonge Street
18th Floor
P O Box 2431
Toronto
ON M4P 1E4
416 486 8584
416 484 6821
info@ccnm.edu

Canadian Naturopathic Association
4174 Dundas Street W
Suite 304
Etobicoke
M8X 1X3
416 233 1043
416 233 2924

New Zealand

New Zealand Society of Naturopaths
P O Box 90–170
Auckland
09 846 6684
09 846 6152

South Africa

Naturopath Association
011 622 6967

UK

British College of Naturopathy and Osteopathy
Frazer House
6 Netherhall Gardens
London NW3 5RR
0171 435 6464
0171 431 3630

General Council and Register of Naturopaths
Goswell House
2 Goswell Road
Street
Somerset BA16 0JG
01458 840072
01458 840075

USA

American Association of Naturopathic Physicians
601 Valley Street
Suite 105
Seattle
WA 98109
206 289 0126
206 298 0129

American Naturopathic Association
1413 King Street
First Floor
Washington
DC 20005
202 682 7352
202 289 2027

National College of Naturopathic Medicine
11231 Southeast Market Street
Portland
OR 97216
503 255 4860

Osteopathy

Australia

Australian Osteopathic Association
Federal Office
P O Box 699
Turramurra 2074
029 449 4799
029 449 6587
aoa@tpgi.com.au

Canada

British Columbia Osteopathic Association
461 Martin Street
Penticton
BC V2A 5L1
604 492 2611

Canadian College of Osteopathy
39 Alvin Avenue
Toronto
ON M4T 2A7
416 323 1465
416 323 1864

Canadian Osteopathic Association
575 Waterloo Street
London
ON N6B 2R2
519 439 5521

South Africa

Osteopathic Society
011 442 9393

UK

General Osteopathic Council
Premier House
10 Greycoat Place
London SW1P 1SB
0171 799 2442
0171 799 2332
gosc@osteopathy.org.uk

USA

American Academy of Osteopathy
3500 De Pauw Boulevard
Suite 1080
Indianapolis
IN 46268
317 879 1881

American Osteopathic Association
142 East Ontario Street
Chicago
IL 60611
312 280 5800

The Cranial Academy
8606 Allisonville Road
Suite 130
Indianapolis
IN 46250
317 594 0411
cranacad@aol.com

Pilates

Australia

Australian Pilates Method Association
P O Box 27
Mosman
NSW 2088
029 929 8807

Pilates Institute of Australia
2 George Street
Sydney
NSW 2000
029 267 8223
029 267 8226

South Africa

Pilates Body Control
Suite 151
Private Bag X3036
Postnet Paarl 7620
021 863 3337
021 863 3337

UK

Pilates Foundation
80 Camden Road
London E17 7NF
07071 81859

USA

The Physicalmind Institute
1807 Second Street
Suite 47
Santa Fe
NM 87505
505 988 1990
505 988 2837

Pilates Guild
890 Broadway
Suite 201
New York
NY 10023-1786
212 875 0189
212 769 2368
Mrpilates@aol.com

Polarity therapy

UK

British Polarity Council
Monomonk House
27 Old Gloucester Street
London WC1N 3XX
01483 417714

Federation of Polarity Training
7 Nunney Close
Golden Valley
Cheltenham
Gloucestershire
GL51 0TU

USA

American Polarity Therapy Association
2888 Bluff Street
Suite 149
Boulder
CO 80301
303 545 2080
303 545 2161
hg@polaritytherapy.org

Psychodrama

UK

British Association of Dramatherapists
5 Sunnydale Villas
Durlston Road
Swanage
Dorset BH19 2HY

Hoewell International Centre for Psychodrama
North Walk
Lynton
North Devon EX35 6HJ
01598 753754
01598 753555
Hoewell@zambula.demon.co.uk

Oxford Psychodrama Group
8 Rahere Road
Cowley
Oxford OX4 3QG
01865 715055

USA

American Society of Group Psychotherapy & Psychodrama
301 N Harrison Street
Suite 508
Princeton
NJ 08540
609 452 1339
609 936 1569

National Association for Drama Therapy
44 Taylor Place
Branford
CT 06405
203 481 1161
203 483 7373

Psychodrama Training Institute
19th West 34th Street
Penthouse, New York
NY 10001
212 947 7111
212 239 0948

Qigong (Chi Kung)

Australia

Qigong Association of Australia
458 White Horse Road
Surrey Hills
VI 3127
039 836 6961

UK

Tse Qigong Centre
P O Box 116
Manchester M20 3YN
0161 929 4485
0161 292 4489

USA

International Institute of Medical Qigong
P O Box 52144
Pacific Grove
CA 93950
831 646 9399
831 646 0535

National Qigong (Chi Kung) Association
571 Selby Avenue
St Paul
MN 55102
888 218 7788
612 291 7779
webmaster@nqa.org

Qigong Human Life Research Foundation
P O Box 5327
Cleveland
Ohio 44101
216 475 4712

Qigong Institute
East West Academy of Healing Arts
450 Sutter Street
Suite 916
San Francisco
CA 94108
415 788 2227

Yan Xin Qigong Educational Centre
901 N Prospect Avenue
Champaign
IL 61820

Radionics

UK

Confederation of Radionics and Radiesthesic Organizations
Radionics and Radiesthesia Trust
Wincanton BA9 8EH
01963 32651

Radionic Association
Baerlein House
Goose Green
Deddington
Banbury
Oxfordshire OX15 0SZ
01869 338852

Reflexology

Australia

Reflexology Association of Australia
P O Box 366
Cammeray
NSW 2062
024 721 4752
029 631 3287

Canada

Ontario College of Reflexology
P O Box 220
New Liskeard
ON P0J 1P0
705 647 5354
705 647 0719

Reflexology Association of Canada
11 Glen Cameron Road
Unit 4 Thornhill
ON L3T 4N3
905 889 5900

Ireland

Irish Reflexologists' Institute
4 Ruskin Park
Lisburn
County Antrim
01846 677806
kathyrea@home2.dnet.co.uk

Society of Reflexologists of Ireland
41 Parkfield, New Ross
County Wexford
051 422209
footman@tinet.ie

New Zealand

New Zealand Institute of Reflexologists Inc
253 Mount Albert Road
Mount Roskill
Auckland

USEFUL INFORMATION

New Zealand Reflexology Association
P O Box 31084
Auckland 9
064 9486 1918
064 9489 2916

South Africa

South African Academy of Reflexology
9a 11th Avenue
Homestead Road
Rivonia 2128
011 803 1552
011 803 5946

South African Reflexology Society
P O Box 1780
New Germany 3620
031 705 5566
031 705 5762

UK

Association of Reflexologists
27 Old Gloucester Street
London WC1N 3XX
0870 567 3320
aor@reflexology.org

British Reflexology Association
Monks Orchard
Whitborne
Worcester WR6 5RB
01886 821207
01886 821207

Holistic Association of Reflexologists
Holistic Healing Centre
92 Sheering Road
Old Harlow
Essex CM17 0JW
01279 429060

International Federation of Reflexologists
78 Edridge Road
Croydon
Surrey CR0 1EF
0181 667 9458

International Institute of Reflexology
Reflexology Centre
32 Priory Road
Portbury
Bristol BS20 9TH
01275 373359

Reflexologists Society
39 Presbury Road
Cheltenham
Gloucestershire GL52 2PT
01242 512601

Scottish Institute of Reflexology
17 Cainwell Avenue
Mastrick
Aberdeen AB16 5SH
01224 697309

USA

International Institute of Reflexology
P O Box 12642
St Petersburg
FL 33733–2642
813 343 4811

New England Association of Reflexology
P O Box 1718
Onset
MA 02558
508 291 1729

Nevada Reflexology Organization
5025 S Eastern Avenue
P O Box 16–357
Las Vegas
NA 89119–2369
702 795 7300
702 795 7201

New York State Reflexology Association
1492 Sweeney Street
North Tonawanda
NY 14120
716 693 3068

Reflexology Association of America
4012 South Rainbow Boulevard
PO Box K585
Las Vegas
NV 89103–2059
702 871 9522

Reflexology Association of California
P O Box 641156
Los Angeles
CA 90064

Reiki

Canada

Atlantic Usui Reiki Association
RR Apartment 2 Stewiacke
Nova Scotia
B0N 2J0
jsettle@atcon.com

Canadian Reiki Association
PO Box 40026
RPO Marlee
Toronto
ON M6B 4K4
416 242 6819 (fax)
lhcaplan@compuserve.com

Ottawa Area Reiki Centre
3428 Woodroffe Avenue
Nepean
ON K3J 4G5
613 823 7113

Reiki Training Centre of Canada
PO Box 3294
Sherwood Park
AL T8A 2A6
403 467 6621

Traditional Japanese Reiki Association
Aurora Holistic Centre
4556–99 Street
Edmonton
AL T6E 5H5
403 437 5481
tjreiki@connect.ab.ca

Netherlands

Reiki Alliance Europe
Honthorstraat 40 111 1071 DG
Amsterdam
31 20 6719276
31 20 6711736
100125.4662@compuserve.com

New Zealand

Reiki New Zealand Inc
PO Box 60–226
Titirangi
Auckland
reiki@ihug.co.nz

UK

Reiki Association
Cornbrook Bridge House
Clee Hill
Ludlow
Shropshire SY8 3QQ
01584 891197
01584 891197
KateJones@reikiassociation.org.uk

Reiki Kyokai Usui Shiki Ryoho
218 Osborne Road
Jesmond
Newcastle upon Tyne NE2 3LB
0191 281 7442
106622.1776@compuserve.com

USA

American Reiki Master Association
Omega Dawn Sanctuary of the Healing Arts
PO Box 130
Lake City
FL 32056–0130
904 755 9638
904 755 9638
arma@atlantic.net

International Association of Reiki Professionals
PO Box 481
Winchester
MA 01890
781 729 3530
781 721 7306
info@iarp.org

International Center for Reiki Training
21421 Hilltop Street
Apartment 28
Southfield
MI 48034–1023
248 948 8112
248 948 9534
center@reiki.org

International Reiki Healing Association
2261 Market Street
Suite 238
San Francisco
CA 94114
415 771 4991

Northwest Reiki Institute
PO Box 342
Langley
WA 98260
360 221 6143
360 221 6961

Reiki Alliance
PO Box 41
Cataldo
ID 83810–1041
208 682 4848
74051.3471@compuserve.com

Reiki Center for Healing Arts
1764 Hamlet Street
San Mateo
CA 94403
413 345 7666

Reiki Cooperative
2164 Philip Drive
Bensalem
PA 19020
215 638 1329
Myrium@aol.com

Reiki Healers' Association
5462 Noyestar Road
E Hardwick
VT 05836–9826
802 533 2527
pemadolk@plainfield.bypass.com

Reiki Healing Connection
633 Isaac Frye Hwy
Wilton
NH 03086
603 654 2787
603 654 2771
Reiki@jlc.net

Reiki Healing Institute
449 Sante Fe Drive
Apartment 303
Ensinitas
CA 92024
619 436 6875

Reiki Outreach International
PO Box 609
Fair Oaks
CA 95628
916 863 6464

Reiki Plus Institute
130 Ridge Road
Celina
TN 38551
931 243 3712
931 243 4657
reikiplus@twlakes.net

Rolfing

Australia

Rolf Institute
Pacific Basin Branch
P O Box 161
Paddington
NSW 2021

Germany
European Rolfing Association
Kapuziner Strasse 25
D 80337 Munchen
089 396 802
089 392 583
rolfingeurope@compuserve.com

UK
Rolfing Institute
P O Box 14793
London SW1V 2WB

USA
Guild for Structural Integration
P O Box 1559
Boulder
CO 80306
303 447 0122
303 447 0180
gsi@rolfguild.org

Rolf Institute of Structural Integration
205 Canyon Boulevard
Boulder
CO 80302-4920
303 449 5903
303 449 5978
RolfInst@rolf.org

Shiatsu

Australia
Shiatsu Therapy Association of Australia
PO Box 1
Balaclava 3183
039 530 0067
039 530 0067

New Zealand
European Shiatsu School
55 Te Manuao Road
Otaki
636 364 6504

UK
British School of Shiatsu Do
6 Erskine Road
London NW3 3AJ
0171 483 3776 (fax)

European Shiatsu Network
Highbanks
Lockeridge
Marlborough
Wiltshire SN8 4TQ
01672 861362
01672 831459

Shiatsu Society
31 Pullman Lane
Godalming
Surrey GU7 1XY
01483 860771
01483 860771

USA
School of Shiatsu and Massage
PO Box 889
Middletown
CA 95461
707 987 3801
707 987 9638

Sound therapy

Australia
Health and Education Association for Research into Sound (HEARS)
3 Coutts Place
Melba
Canberra
ACT 2615
026 259 1364
026 258 5530
kdistel@pcug.org.au

UK
Cymatics Ltd
Bretforton Hall Clinic
Main Street
Bretforton
Evesham
Worcestershire WR11 5JH
01386 830537
01386 830918

Inner Sound
8 Elms Avenue
London N10 2JP
0181 444 4855

Light and Sound Therapy Centre
90 Queen Elizabeth's Walk
London N16 5UQ
0181 880 1269
0181 880 1260
light-sound@ait-help.demon.co.uk

USA
Sound Healers Association
P O Box 2240
Boulder CO 80306
303 443 8181
303 443 6023

Tomatis Center
3700 M Diablo Boulevard
Suite 300
Lafayette
CA 94596
510 284 8431
510 284 8431

T'ai chi

Australia
Taoist T'ai Chi Society of Western Australia
PO Box 824
Freemantle
WA 6160

Canada
Taoist T'ai Chi Society of Canada
1376 Bathurst Street
Toronto
ON M5R 3J1
416 656 2110
416 654 3937

UK

Taoist T'ai Chi Centre
Bounstead Road
Blackheath
Colchester
Essex CO2 0DE
01206 576167
01206 572269

USA

Taoist T'ai Chi Society of USA
1310 North Monroe Street
Tallahassee
Florida 32303
904 224 5438

Traditional Chinese Medicine

Canada

Academy of Classical Oriental Sciences
420 Railway Street
Nelson
BC V1L 1H3
250 352 5587
250 352 3458
acos@acos.org

Chinese Medicine and Acupuncture Association of Canada
154 Wellington Street
London
ON N6B 2K8
519 642 1970

China

Fujian University of Traditional Chinese Medicine
282 Wusi Road
Fuzhou
Fujian
People's Republic of China
0591 7842528
0591 7842524

South Africa

021 761 7732

USA

American Association of Oriental Medicine
433 Front Street
Catasauqua
PA 18032
610 266 1433
610 264 2768

American College of Traditional Chinese Medicine
455 Arkansas Street
San Francisco
CA 94107
415 282 7600
415 282 0856

American Oriental Bodywork Therapy Association
Glendale Executive Campus
Suite 500
1000 White Horse Road
Voorhees
NJ 08043
609 782 1616
609 782 1653

Atlantic Institute of Oriental Medicine
1057 SE 17 Street
Fort Lauderdale
FL 33316–2116
954 463 3888

California Society for Oriental Medicine
12926 Riverside Drive
Suite B
Sherman Oaks
CA 91423
818 789 2468
818 981 2766

Chinese Healing Arts Center
73–3 Great Plain Road
Danbury
CT 06811
914 687 0988
914 687 0988
QiHealer@aol.com

East West Academy of Healing Arts
561 Berkeley Avenue
Menlo Park
CA 94025

Emperor's College of Traditional Oriental Medicine
1807B Wilshire Boulevard
Santa Monica
CA 90403
310 453 8300

International Institute of Chinese Medicine
4600 Montgomery Boulevard NE 1–1
Albuquerque
NM 87109
505 880 9778
505 880 1775
panda@thuntek.net

Institute for Traditional Medicine
2017 SE Hawthorne Boulevard
Portland
OR 97214
itm@europa.com

National Certification Commission for Acupuncture and Oriental Medicine
11 Canal Center Plaza
Suite 300
Alexandria
VA 22314
703 548 9004
703 548 9079

Oregon College of Oriental Medicine
10525 SE Cherry Blossom Drive
Portland OR 97216
503 253 3443
503 253 2701

Trager bodywork

UK
Trager Association UK
64 Wilbury Road
Hove
Sussex BN3 3PY

USA
Florida Institute of Psychophysical Integration
Quantum Balance
5837 Mariner Drive
Tampa
FL 33609–3411
813 286 2273
813 287 2870

Trager Institute
21 Locust Avenue
Mill Valley
CA 94941–2806
415 388 2688
415 388 2710
admin@trager.com

Visualization

USA
Academy for Guided Imagery
PO Box 2070
Mill Valley
CA 94942
800 726 2070

Yoga

Australia
Australian Institute of Yoga Therapy
7/71 Ormond Road
Elwood
VIC 3184
039 525 6951
yogather@hotkey.net.au

Yoga Synergy
P O Box 9
Waverley 2024
029 389 7399
029 389 7238
physio@yogasynergy.com.au

Canada
Healing Through Yoga
Box 834
Kamloops
BC V2C 5M8
250 374 2514
800 667 4550

Yoga Association of Alberta
11759 Groat Road
Edmonton
AB T5M 3K6
403 453 8673
403 453 8553

Yoga Center Toronto
2428 Yonge Street
Toronto
ON M4P 2H4
416 482 1334
416 482 2953

Yoga Meditation Center of Regina
30 Plainsview Drive
Regina
SK S4S 6K3
306 586 4133
306 525 6757

South Africa

Yoga Teachers Fellowship of South Africa
P O Box 7598
Bonaero Park 1622
011 787 0884

UK

British School of Yoga
The Old Vicarage
Clawton
Nr Holsworthy
Devon EX22 6PS
01409 271432

British Wheel of Yoga
1 Hamilton Place
Boston Road
Sleaford
Lincolnshire NG34 7ES
01529 306851

Iyengar Yoga Institute
223a Randolph Avenue
London W9 1NL
0171 624 3080

Yoga Centre
16 Canning Street
Edinburgh EH3 8EG
0131 221 9697
0131 221 9697

Yoga for Health Foundation
Ickwell Bury
Northill
Biggleswade
Bedfordshire SG18 9EF
01767 627271

USA

American Institute of Vedic Studies
P O Box 8357
Santa Fe
NM 87504
505 983 9385
vedicinst@aol.com

American Yoga Association
P O Box 19986
Sarasota
FL 34276
941 927 4977
941 921 9844
YOGAmerica@aol.com

International Association of Yoga Therapists
20 Sunnyside Avenue
Suite A–243
Mill Valley
CA 94941-1928
415 332 2478
415 381 0876

International Yoga Therapy & Ayurveda Institute
111 Elm Street
Suite 103, Worcester
MA 01609
508 755 3744
ayurveda@hotmail.com

**Iyengar Yoga National
  Association of the USA**
544 Orme Cir NE
Atlanta
GA 30306–3652
404 874 5082

**World Union of Yoga/
  International Association
  of Yoga**
Yoga Therapy Center
120-A Westbourne Terrace
Brookline
MA 02446
617 739 1146
yogimuk@banet.net

Yoga Research Center
P O Box 1386
Lower Lake
CA 95457
707 928 9898
707 928 4738
yogaresrch@aol.com

FURTHER READING

Alexander, F M, *The Use of the Self*, Gollancz, 1985
Alvin, Juliette, *Music Therapy*, Stainer & Bell Ltd, 1966. Revised 1983 and 1991
Angelo, Jack, *Spiritual Healing*, Element, 1991
Bates, W H, *Better Eyesight Without Glasses*, Holt, Rinehart and Winston, 1919, (many reprints currently available)
Brooke, Elisabeth, *A Woman's Book of Herbs*, Women's Press, 1992 (reprinted 1999)
Brown, Loulou, *Working in Complementary and Alternative Medicine: A Career Guide*, Kogan Page, 1994
Craze, Richard, *Teach Yourself Alexander Technique*, Hodder & Stoughton, 1996
Craze, Richard, with Jen T'ieh, *Teach Yourself Traditonal Chinese Medicine*, Hodder & Stoughton, 1998
Culpeper, Nicholas, *English Physician and Complete Herbal*, first published 1653, (many reprints currently available)
Dougans, Inge, *Reflexology: A Practical Introduction*, Element, 1998
Ernst, Edzard, *Complementary Medicine: An Objective Appraisal*, Butterworth, 1996
Feldenkrais, M, *Awareness Through Movement: health exercises for personal growth*, Harper & Row, 1972
Fulder, Stephen, *The Handbook of Alternative and Complementary Medicine*, Vermilion, 1996 (third edition)
Gerson, Scott, *Ayurveda: The Ancient Indian Healing Art*, Element, 1992
Goldstein, Joseph, *Transforming the Mind, Healing the World*, Paulist Press, 1994
Hill, Ann, (ed) *A Visual Encyclopedia of Unconventional Medicine*, New English Library, 1979
Huxley, Aldous, *The Art of Seeing*, Penguin, 1943

Jackson, Adam J, *Eye Signs*, Thorsons, 1995

Jamil, Tanvir, *Complementary Medicine A Practical Guide*, Butterworth, 1997

Jarmey, Chris, *Shiatsu*, Thorsons, 1992

Kermani, Dr Kai, *Autogenic Training*, Souvenir, 1999 (second edition)

Krämar, Dietmar, *New Bach Flower Therapies*, Healing Arts Press, 1989

Leibowitz, Judith and Connington, Bill, *The Alexander Technique*, Souvenir Press, 1991 (first British edition)

Lockie, Dr Andrew, *The Family Guide to Homoeopathy*, Hamish Hamilton, 1990

Marti, James, with Hine, Andrea, *The Alternative Health & Medicine Encyclopaedia*, Gale Research Inc, 1995

McNamara, Sheila and Dr Song Xuan Ke, *Traditional Chinese Medicine*, Hamish Hamilton, 1995

Mitchell, Stuart, *Naturopathy: Understanding the Healing Power of Nature*, Element, 1998

Mole, Peter, *Acupuncture: energy balancing for body, mind & spirit*, Element, 1992

Nash, Barbara, *A–Z of Complementary Health*, Ward Lock, 1995

Norman, Laura with Cowan, Thomas, *The Reflexology Handbook*, Piatkus, 1989

Oxford Reference, *Concise Medical Dictionary*, Oxford University Press, 1990 (third edition)

Peiffer, Vera, *Principles of Hypnotherapy*, Thorsons, 1996

Price, Shirley, *Practical Aromatherapy: How to Use Essential Oils to Restore Vitality*, Thorsons, 1987 (second edition)

Reader's Digest Family Guide to Alternative Medicine, Reader's Digest Association, 1991

River, Lindsay and Gillespie, Sally *The Knot of Time*, Women's Press, 1987

Ridder-Patrick, Jane, *A Handbook of Medical Astrology*, Penguin, 1990

Robinson, Lynne, and Thomson, Gordon, *Body Control The Pilates Way*, Pan Books, 1998

Rowlands, Barbara, *The Which? Guide to Complementary Medicine*, Consumers' Association, 1977

Shreve, Dr Caroline M, *The Alternative Dictionary of Symptoms and Cures*, Century, 1986

Smyth, Angela, *The Complete Encyclopaedia of Natural Health*, Thorsons, 1997

Stalmatski, Alexander, *Freedom from Asthma: Buteyko's Revolutionary Treatment*, Kyle Cathie, 1977
Svoboda, Robert, *Ayurveda: Life Health and Longevity*, Penguin, 1992
Vithoulkas, George, *Homoeopathy*, Thorsons, 1985
Warrier, Gopi and Gunawant, Deepika, *The Complete Illustrated Guide to Ayurveda*, Element Books, 1997
Watson, Donald, *A Dictionary of Mind and Body*, Andre Deutsch, 1995
Webb, Dr Peter, *The Family Encyclopaedia of Homoeopathic Remedies*, Robinson, 1997
Weil, Andrew, *Natural Health, Natural Medicine*, Warner Books, 1995
Whichello Brown, Denise, *Teach Yourself Aromatherapy*, Hodder & Stoughton, 1996
Wildwood, Christine, *Flower Remedies: Natural Healing with Flower Essences,* Element, 1992
Woodham, Anne and Peters, Dr David, *Encyclopedia of Complementary Medicine*, Dorling Kindersley, 1997

INDEX

Abrams, Dr Albert 122
acupoints 27, 30, 130
acupressure 5, 15, 18, 21, 22, 23, 27–8, 137, 148, 149, 150, 151, 152, 153, 154
  organizations 161
acupuncture 5, 7, 18, 22, 23, 27, 28–31, 147, 148, 149, 150, 151, 152, 153, 154
  needles 30–1
  organizations 161–3
Alexander, Frederick Matthias 32
Alexander Technique 10–11, 14, 17, 18, 22, 31-5, 52, 56, 147, 150, 151, 152, 153
  organizations 163–4
allopathic medicine *see* orthodox medicine
alternative medicine
  cost 20
  growth of 7–8
  in Australia 5–6
  in New Zealand 6
  in South Africa 6
  in the West 5–8
  in UK 6–7
  in USA 7
  lack of proof of effectiveness 14
  what it is 3–5
alternative remedies 9–10

anthroposophical medicine 18, 35–6
  organizations 165
aromatherapy 5, 7, 11, 15, 17, 18, 19, 21, 22, 23, 36–41, 98, 147, 148, 149, 150, 151, 152, 153, 154
  massage 39
  organizations 165–7
art therapy 6, 16, 18, 21, 41-2, 147, 148, 150, 152, 153
  organizations 167
autogenic training 18, 22, 42–4, 52, 150, 151, 153
  organizations 168
autonomic nervous system 14, 52, 103
autonomic responses 51, 52, 89
autosuggestion 18, 44–5, 147, 152
Ayurveda 5, 7, 11, 18, 45–7, 118, 147, 148, 149, 154
  organizations 168–9
Ayurvedic remedies 9, 47

Bach, Dr Edward 69
Bach flower remedies 5, 21, 69–70, 147, 150, 151, 154
  organizations *see* flower remedies
Bach rescue remedy 10, 70
Bates method 18, 47–9, 149
  organizations, 169–70

Bates, William 48
bioenergetics 18, 49–50, 52, 151
  organizations 170
biofeedback training 5, 11, 14, 18, 22, 50–3, 147, 148, 150, 151, 152, 153, 154
  organizations 170–1
biorhythms 18, 53–4
Braid, Dr James 89
breathing and relaxation 16, 17, 18, 21, 22, 23, 47, 52, 55–7, 103, 147, 148, 149, 150, 151, 152, 153
Buteyko, K P 58
Buteyko method 18, 57–8, 147
  organization 171

chi kung *see* qigong
Chinese herbal medicine 5, 6, 11, 18, 21, 22, 23, 75–8, 137, 147, 148, 149, 150, 152, 153
  organizations 176
chiropractic 6, 7, 10–11, 14, 18, 19, 21, 22, 59–63, 98, 147, 148, 150, 151, 152, 154
  organizations 171–3
colour therapy 18, 19, 63–4, 147
  organization 173
Confederation of Healing Organizations' Code of Conduct 72–3
conventional medicine *see* orthodox medicine
Coué, Emile 44
cranial osteopathy 17, 21, 23, 115, 148, 149, 150, 151, 152, 154
  organizations *see* osteopathy
creative therapies 18
crystal and gem therapies 18, 64–5
  organizations 173
cymatic therapy 131

dance therapy 18, 21, 23, 65–6, 147, 150
  organizations 173–4
de la Warr, George 122
doshas 45, 47
Downing, George 98

essential oils 36–41
exercise 16
exercise therapies 18

fascia 73, 74, 128
Feldenkrais, Dr Moshe 67
Feldenkrais method 18, 67–8
  organizations 174
finding the right therapist 12, 19
Fitzgerald, Dr William 123
flotation therapy 17, 18, 23, 68–9
  organizations 174
flower remedies 5, 9, 18, 19, 69–70
  organizations 175
further reading 205–7

Gattefossé, Professor René-Maurice 37
'general' organizations 157–60
Gerson, Scott 45
Goodhart, Dr George 96
Gunawant, Deepika 45

Hahnemann, Samuel 84
hatha yoga *see* yoga
healing 7, 14, 18, 19, 70–3, 152, 154
  organizations 175–6
healthy eating 15–16

INDEX

Heller, Joseph 73
Hellerwork 18, 19, 73–5
  organization 176
herbal medicine 7, 11, 18
herbal medicine – Chinese *see* Chinese herbal medicine
herbal medicine – Western *see* Western herbal medicine
herbal remedies 6, 9, 77–8, 81–3
Hippocrates 59, 109
holistic medicine 3–5
homeostasis 4, 70, 78, 109
homeostatic processes 11, 101, 103
homoeopathic remedies 6, 9, 86
homoeopathy 5, 6, 7, 11, 14, 18, 21, 22, 23, 83–7, 147, 148, 149, 150, 151, 152, 153, 154
  organizations 178–9
hydrotherapy 18, 22, 23, 87–8, 148, 149, 150, 151, 152, 153, 154
  organizations 179–80
hypnosis 11, 89
hypnotherapy 18, 22, 89–92, 148, 152, 153, 154
  organizations 180–1

Ingham Eunice, 123
iridology 18, 93–5
  organizations, 181–2

Jensen, Dr Bernard 93

Kamiya, Dr Joe 51
keeping doctor informed 20
ki *see* Qi
kinesiology 18, 95–6, 137, 150, 153
  organizations 182

Laban, Rudolph 65

lifestyle 9, 13, 15–17
light therapy 18, 97–8, 151, 153
  organizations 183
Lilly, John C 68
Ling, Henrik 98
Lowen, Dr Alexander 49

McTimoney chiropractic 60, 63
  organizations *see* chiropractic
McTimoney-Corley chiropractic 60, 63
  organizations *see* chiropractic
manipulative/touch therapies 18, 19
massage 6, 11, 13, 17, 18, 19, 21, 22, 98–101, 147, 148, 149, 150, 151, 152, 153, 154
  organizations 183–4
Maury, Marguerite 37
medical astrology 18, 101–2
  organizations 185
meditation 14, 17, 18, 22, 23, 47, 52, 55, 56, 102–5, 147, 149, 150, 151, 152, 153
  organizations 185–6
Mentastics 139
meridians 30, 31, 95, 121, 135
metamorphic technique 18, 105–7
  organizations 186
mind/spirit therapies 18
Moreno, Jacob 119
moxibustion 30
music therapy 17, 18, 19, 22, 107–8, 149, 151, 153
  organizations 186–7

naturopathy 6, 7, 16, 18, 21, 22, 23, 108–12, 147, 148, 149, 150, 151, 152, 153, 154
  organizations 187–8

oral therapies 18
orthodox medicine 3, 5, 9, 135
　limitations 8
　problems best treated by 14–15
orthodox practitioners 20–1, 43
osteopathy 5, 6, 11, 14, 18, 19, 22, 23, 98, 112–16, 150, 151, 152, 153, 154
　organizations, 188–9
Outline of Materia Medica 75

Palmer, Bartlett J 59–60
Palmer, Daniel David 59
Pilates 14, 18, 23, 116–17, 149, 154
　organizations 189–90
Pilates, Joseph H 116
polarity therapy 18, 118–19, 153, 154
　organizations 190
prana 45, 59, 109, 135
psychodrama 18, 119–20, 147, 148
　organizations 190–1

Qi 27, 28, 29, 30, 31, 55, 59, 75, 109, 120, 121, 127, 129, 132, 135
qigong 16, 18, 56, 120–1, 150, 151
　organizations, 191–2

radionics 14, 18, 122–3
　organizations 192
reductionist principles 3
reflexology 15, 18, 19, 21, 22, 23, 123–7, 147, 149, 151, 153
　organizations 192–4
reiki 18, 127–8, 147, 150, 151
　organizations 194–6
remedies over the counter 9–10
Rolf, Dr Ida 73, 128

Rolfing 14, 18, 22, 128–9, 150
　organizations, 196–7

St John, Robert 105–6
Schultz, Dr Johannes 43
shiatsu 18, 129–30, 137, 147, 151, 153
　organizations 197–8
Shi-zhen, Li 75
sleep 16
sound therapy 18, 131–2, 153
　organizations, 198
Steiner, Rudolph 35
Still, Andrew Taylor 112–13
Stone, Dr Randolph 118
Swedish massage *see* massage
Svoboda, Robert 45

t'ai chi 16, 18, 56, 132–4, 137, 150, 152, 153
　organizations, 198–9
Takata, Hawaio 127
TCM *see* Traditional Chinese Medicine
therapists
　importance of fully qualified 12
　respect for whole individual 13
Traditional Chinese Medicine 5, 7, 27, 28, 29, 55, 75, 76, 95, 120, 129, 130, 132, 134–7
　organizations 199–200
Trager bodywork 18, 19, 137–9
　organizations 201
Trager, Dr Milton 138
transcendental meditation 55, 103

Usi, Dr Mikao 127

Valnet, Dr Jean 37
visualization 11, 17, 18, 21, 44, 52, 56, 139–41, 147, 153
  organization 201
von Peczely 93

Warrier, Gopi 45
water therapies 18
Western herbal medicine 5, 6, 11, 18, 21, 22, 23, 78–83, 147, 148, 149, 150, 151, 152, 153, 154
  organizations 177–8

yang 135
yin 135
yoga 14, 17, 18, 22, 23, 47, 55, 56, 103, 118, 141–4, 147, 149, 151, 152, 153, 154
  organizations 201–3
Yogi, Maharishi Mahesh 103